MY LIFE WITHOUT l

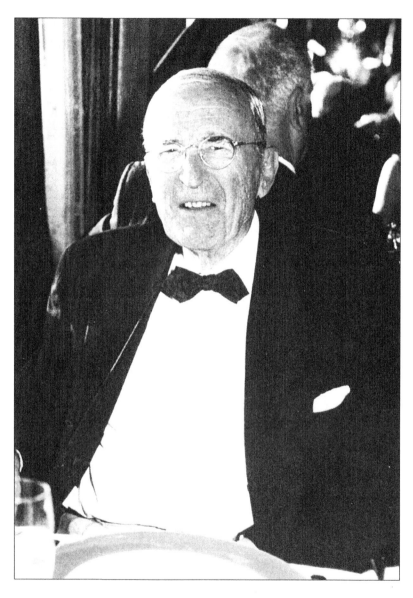

Wolfgang Lutz celebrating his 90th birthday at the Athenaeum

My Life Without Bread
Dr Lutz at 90

Valerie Bracken

JUST PERHAPS?

EDINBURGH

Also by Valerie Bracken
Uncle Wolfi's Secret

Copyright © Valerie Bracken, 2014
All rights reserved
The moral right of the author has been asserted

First published in Great Britain in 2014 by
JUST PERHAPS?
www.justperhaps.co.uk

ISBN 978-0-9926944-1-8

A catalogue record for this book is available
from the British Library

Typeset and designed by Zebedee Design

Printed by CreateSpace

ACKNOWLEDGEMENTS

First and foremost, I would like to express my gratitude to the late Dr Wolfgang Lutz for all that I have learnt from him over the years or that he has inspired me to learn.

I would like to thank Dr Erdmuthe Idris for her kind permission to include material from the books by Dr Lutz that were published by INFORMED and Selecta-Verlag. I also thank Monica Groves for her kind permission to use her photograph of Dr Lutz, Helen Lutz for supplying the frontispiece and Christian Allan for his preface.

Finally, I would like to thank all those who have given me help, support and advice during the long gestation period of this book, including reading and commenting on the various stages of the manuscript: Dr Lutz himself and his wife Helen, Dr W Yellowlees and the late Barry Groves and his wife Monica. I thank, too, my close friends and family for their interest, patience and encouragement, and especially my husband Mark.

To all those who stand to benefit from
the information contained in this book

JUST PERHAPS?

aims to celebrate the work of pioneering doctors
who have dedicated their lives to an aspect of medical
practice that lies outside the mainstream yet
which – just perhaps – has something of
vital importance to offer us.

CONTENTS

A BRILLIANT ACHIEVEMENT

My journey to seek the truth behind nutrition and its relationship to health led me directly to the brilliant lifetime achievement that Dr Wolfgang Lutz brought to the world. Wolfgang Lutz was one of the pioneers of low carbohydrate nutrition and his discoveries were no small feat. Through the work that he did with his patients starting back in the late 1950's, and through his theories, observations and studies, Dr Lutz presented the world with simple tools to significantly reduce the disease burden of modern times. He was ahead of his time in this regard and, at the time, the world wasn't quite ready.

I had the great privilege to meet Wolfgang Lutz and to co-author a book with him. The path that led me to this started early in the 1990's. Well before I met Wolfgang, I was already deeply interested in the link between nutrition and disease, the prevailing assumption being that fat and cholesterol were the food components that caused so many of those diseases we term diseases of civilization, such as cancer, heart disease and Crohn's. Trained as a chemist and biochemist, I began my search through the medical and nutritional literature with open eyes, untainted by prevailing dogma. As I looked into the theories and published literature on this subject, it was clear that, though it was 'known' by almost everyone to be true, there was neither any real proof nor even any quality data to support the fat hypothesis.

So how did I first learn about Wolfgang's work? Serendipity! When I was a graduate student of chemistry at the University of Pacific in California, I visited a friend at the University of

California Davis. There was a book sale at the Davis campus library and I purchased a case of nutrition books without much concern for the specific books in the collection. I briefly read the title of each book and then packed them back in the box. A few years later, as my interest in low carbohydrate nutrition grew, I recalled that I had a book on this subject in the box of books that I had purchased at the Davis library sale. I still remember that day in Western Massachusetts when I pulled out the English translation of Wolfgang's German book *Leben Ohne Brot.* It was called *Dismantling a Myth: The Role of Fat and Carbohydrates in our Diet* and I read it in just a few days. And that was it! What I read astonished me. It substantiated the value of low-carbohydrate nutrition in reducing and treating non-infectious disease and was the greatest set of data and studies on the subject that I had seen at the time. This was in 1995 and, enthusiastically, I spent many months piecing together additional parts of the puzzle from a biochemical perspective and researched the most recent material on nutrition and disease. I also began to adopt a low-carbohydrate diet myself.

I was so excited by Wolfgang's work and the plethora of recent data that supported the basic principle of low carbohydrate nutrition that I decided to contact Wolfgang Lutz in person. This I did and a year or two later we met in Washington D C and then in Salzburg. We decided to find a publisher in the US to re-release his English book *Dismantling a Myth.* I was subsequently in contact with Keats Publishing; there was no interest in a re-release in the US but I was asked to help edit their scientific publications to make them more reader friendly to lay people. I did this for a number of months, after which I told them that what I was really interested in was publishing a book on low-carbohydrate nutrition based on Wolfgang's data. My persistence paid off. After a time, Peter, the editor at Keats Publishing, whom I was working with, suggested that Wolfgang and I write a new book for the US, updated and written for a broader audience to be released by Keats. Thus, in the year 2000, our joint book *Life Without Bread: How a Low-Carbohydrate Diet Can Save Your Life* was spawned.

Today it is very clear that low-carbohydrate nutrition is the correct nutrition for human beings everywhere. There is still resistance but that is fading with every new study that shows the value of this mode of nutrition. A great many people have benefitted from Wolfgang's work, including myself and those close to me. In my opinion, his lifetime of work is deserving of a Nobel Prize. Wolfgang Lutz has provided us with a roadmap to significantly reduce many of our modern diseases by simply reducing the amount of carbohydrates in our diet. There is only one thing left for us to do and that is to learn how to read a map and follow directions.

Christian B Allan, San Francisco 2014

AT NINETY

At the age of ninety, I feel one is entitled to look back! In this book, I look back on my own 'life without bread' and cast an eye over the many years I have been privileged to observe the health-restoring effects of carbohydrate restriction, from the introduction of my diet in the 1950's until the present-day.

Though this book is partly about myself and those I have rubbed shoulders with, most of all it is about the successful implementation of an idea – that our bodies are tuned to the food (and a rhythm) of a bygone age. Nowadays we live and eat very differently and, only when we take this difference on board, do we begin to understand not only why modern notions of good dietary practice are failing us, but also what we can do about it in our daily lives.

My work and my life have been intimately connected. Some of the story has been already told in my other books, especially as regards the use of my diet in the treatment of specific illnesses. Here the focus is rather on how I came to realise the therapeutic possibilities of my diet. I give a more personal account of my work as a doctor and I include some new and some previously untranslated material. The intention is that it should complement my American book *Life without Bread,* which was written jointly with Chris Allan and published in the year 2000. Of course, the real story of my medical work can never be fully put on paper: it is a private story, confidential between me and each person I have treated, with prescriptions tailored as far as possible to individual needs.

How did this book come about? It happened as follows. Some

twelve years ago, the telephone rang in the office of my practice in Salzburg: on the line was an Englishwoman, who was deeply interested in my work. Valerie Bracken had read my book *Dismantling a Myth: the role of fat and carbohydrates in our diet* and was fascinated but critical of its complexity. Could she edit it for me, and so make my message more accessible to the ordinary person seeking guidance as to what to eat to get well and to stay well?

This was a direct challenge to my powers of authorship, and from a complete stranger! However, from this unusual start, there developed a friendship between us. Over the ensuing years, Valerie has become thoroughly conversant with my work, both through my many books and articles, and also through meeting me, talking with me and in prolonged correspondence. Valerie has translated various parts of my work; together we have written prefaces, talks and letters to journals, and also a synopsis of the fourteenth edition of my German book *Leben ohne Brot* (life without bread).

During this time, Valerie and I have had our misunderstandings, have argued – battled even – over details, as I regularly scrutinised and commented on what she wrote. Nevertheless, out of all this, there has eventually emerged a text, which I hope will speak to those who intuitively feel something has gone astray with our modern dietetic thinking. I hope, too, that the detailed descriptions of how I, as a doctor, put my idea of a suitably healing diet into practice with my patients will supply those who follow in my footsteps with the information they need to use my dietary method with understanding.

I congratulate Valerie for bringing together this outline of my life and work from all the various sources I have put at her disposal. It is a praise-worthy exposition of my approach to low carbohydrate nutrition. Naturally, I prefer to write my own books and would love there to be a full and up-to-date English translation of my main book *Leben ohne Brot*. Meanwhile, this present book tells part of the story, and I give it my blessing.

Wolfgang J Lutz, London 2007

PREFACE

As he got older, Wolfgang Lutz, albeit somewhat reluctantly, acknowledged his need for help with his writing. In this, he followed the example of his hero 'Stef'. Vilhjalmur Stefansson was a scholar, a good writer and meticulous about accuracy, yet he expressed his indebtedness to his 'fierce secretary' Olive Wilcox. Blake Donaldson, too, confessed his need for others to arrange his writing and to lop off extraneous material. Dr Lutz was considerably older than either Stef or Donaldson and wanted to write in a language that was not his mother tongue.

Always keeping in the background but too critical to be a ghost, I elected to be this 'fierce secretary', who not just edited his work – Dr Lutz called me Mrs Head Teacher – but also undertook to write for him in English. Hence this present work appearing in the first person, for which I had long had his authorisation – as long, of course, as he checked every word I wrote! The current text was checked and rechecked by Dr Lutz many times. It was completed in 2003 and in 2007 Dr Lutz did give it his blessing. It has since seen only a minor tidying up and the addition of notes.

Wolfgang Lutz never claimed to have said the last word on low carbohydrate nutrition and this work certainly only includes a fraction of his ideas, giving as it does little space to the theoretical side of his work. The result is a somewhat pruned Lutz. *My Life without Bread: Dr Lutz at 90* concentrates on the main premises on which Dr Lutz based his work, on his diet and on the practical side of his medical findings, aiming to describe these as simply and clearly as possible.

I first heard of Wolfgang Lutz when reading the book by Walter Yellowlees *Doctor in the Wilderness*. Writing about the innocence of natural fats as regards causing coronary thrombosis, Dr Yellowlees suggests that our prehistoric forbears lived off the flesh and fat of animals 'since the very dawn of human evolution' and that, according to Dr Lutz, 'our ancestors of this epoch must have relied solely upon game as their food . . .' Solely? Such a barbaric heritage horrified my vegetarian upbringing. I had been interested in nutrition and health for a great many years, but that our insides were therefore adapted primarily to this sort of food was against everything I had ever come across. Yet the idea held a fascination for me; it had a certain ring of truth. Dr Yellowlees then recounts how Dr Lutz tried eating similar fare:

> within a very short time of . . . eating only animal proteins and fats – no carbohydrate at all – the good doctor noted a remarkable improvement in well-being and complete resolution of his dental, digestive and joint troubles.
>
> Yellowlees (1993)

This stopped me in my tracks. I had seen marked improvement in well-being and freedom from pain in joint troubles during my own work as a yoga teacher and remedial masseuse, but complete resolution? The idea was so exciting that I contacted Dr Lutz immediately, and my husband and I then spent many years reading round the topic. In our heart of hearts, we hoped Dr Lutz was mistaken in his view of our ancient diet and also in his proposed treatment of modern ailments. It was not to be. My story *Uncle Wolfi's Secret*, published in 2013 and which I wrote as a tribute to Wolfgang Lutz, features a fictionalised account of this quest.

The above quote highlights the need for accuracy. I admire Dr Yellowlees, who always strives for precision, but was thoroughly relieved to learn that Dr Lutz did not literally mean 'no carbohydrate at all', any more than that he lived for four years on 'only animal proteins and fats', or achieved a 'complete resolution' of his arthritic hips: it was merely his shorthand for 'no cereals', 'predominantly proteins and fats' and the 'restoration of more mobile pain-free hip joints'. Even a 'Life without Bread' should have been a 'Life with Little Bread', as suggested in vain by his good friend Jürgen Schole. Dr Lutz certainly did need an editor and one with a strong will!

So yes, there was a battle between us that went on for many years. This battle was partly about clarity: what did Dr Lutz actually mean by x, y, z? But it was mainly about his beloved epidemiology, on which my background in social science gave me a purchase. My seeming pedantry, my insistence on the accuracy of each detail, both amused and annoyed Dr Lutz. I remember him saying: "I storm ahead and, to make headway, I do not think of little things". Another time he said: "I think like I drive: with my foot down." This splendid self-confidence was coupled with an enduring and endearing sense of fun.

As a physician, his whole demeanour would change: when he was with a patient or talking about a medical problem, Dr Lutz became instantly serious, concerned, compassionate and ready to help. I soon learnt of the impressive healing potential of the Lutz diet: in short, that it could work, and in unexpected ways; that, for some, it offered the only hope of recovery or even improvement; moreover, that it was our best protection against the insidiously detrimental carbohydrate effect. I learnt, too, that it was in no way extraordinary, unpleasant or extreme.

Wolfgang Lutz died on 19 September 2010 at the age of 97 in Graz in his native Austria. Towards the end of his life, Dr Lutz and his work were becoming better known in the United Kingdom and elsewhere. Amongst other marks of recognition, Dr Lutz was included in the Empire Who's Who in 2003-4 and later in the Cambridge Who's Who for 2007-8. In 2004 Dr Lutz received a Certificate from the World Centre for Optimal Nutrition and in 2005 he was awarded an honorary Doctorate of Philosophy by Dublin Metropolitan University, then a Professorship emeritus. In 2007, on January 5th, Wolfgang Lutz was inaugurated in full regalia as Chancellor of that same university.

"Ah, Valerie, I do not need all these honours", he said to me at the time, and then paused: "but for the sake of my work, I am so pleased." However, I know that Wolfgang Lutz was very touched when, on 21st May 2007, he was granted the Freedom of the City of London, a rare distinction for someone from Austria; he was proud to attend the splendid ceremony that was held at the Guildhall that November, inaugurating him as a Freeman of the City. In 2007, Wolfgang Lutz also had the satisfaction that his principal book *Leben ohne Brot* reached its 16th edition after forty years in print. During his lifetime, Dr Lutz wrote several books and over 60 articles on scientific and medical topics. Now, in 2014, *Life without Bread* by Allan & Lutz is still in print after fourteen years.

Though the orthodox medical profession had not exactly welcomed his medical work with open arms, it was widely known in Germany and Austria. Dr Lutz knew many doctors who both practised his diet themselves and who prescribed it to their patients, doing this discreetly; this continued, if quiet, advocacy was heartening to him, as was his success with his own patients. Reflecting on his 'half a life without bread', his comment was: "Contented patients – patients whose symptoms abate and the many who go on to achieve lasting health – are reward enough for a physician".

Dr Lutz liked to socialise; he enjoyed being at his club, dining out or going to the opera. At the same time, he was a deeply private and sensitive person, whose heart lay in his medical work. He had a deep longing that one day the medical profession as a whole would come to realise the invaluable contribution that his diet can make to the healing and prevention of disease – perhaps, with his own work as a signpost?

Valerie Bracken

A TOOL FOR HEALING

Dr Lutz witnessed the wonderful effects of his healing programme, yet cautioned that such a change in diet should be accomplished gradually, especially for men over 35 and women over 60. Dr Lutz felt regular monitoring important and advised those already ill, for instance those with high blood pressure or heart problems or who were overweight or diabetic, to place themselves under the watchful care of their doctor during any period of dietary transition and beyond.

1 BEGINNINGS

This book is the story of a discovery that could bring relief to the suffering of an untold number of people. It is the story of a personal break-through in the field of medicine, a break-through which has already brought relief to many thousands of my patients. I was to find that there is not just a ray of hope but an actual way forward – and a way with little recourse to drugs or surgery – in regard to successfully tackling many of the 'diseases of civilisation'.

The way forward that I am to describe is simple, modest and moderate. It links us with our past in a way that is very relevant to today. During my long medical career, I have been able to confirm in practice that what I propose can help our bodies to run more smoothly and more efficiently, enabling people to be healthier. Amongst other things, I found that it can facilitate better digestion and allow our nervous systems more peace; it can increase our resistance to infection and enhance our ability to cope with other perils that life brings.

Perhaps this improved body functioning contributes in a great measure to the alleviation and amelioration that I have seen over and over again in my medical work with serious illness. Very probably – though this I must leave to time and to others to demonstrate – my method, which is suitable for everyday long-term use, could go a long way in preventing many of these diseases from occurring in the first place. Causation is complex and, obviously, no one measure alone can guarantee immunity against the chronic ailments of our time, nor can one measure offer a panacea in terms of treatment; it may, though, offer a firm foundation on which to build, or rebuild, good health.

The mountains of research and the often conflicting information we are presented with nowadays must only increase the perplexity of the ordinary person trying to get well or to stay well in the modern world. Indeed, to achieve some clarity in this field myself and hence to reach the conclusions I did, there were many questions to ask, many ideas to explore, many clinical observations to make. As a doctor, I have had nearly fifty years experience of using the method I shall describe. I have written other books in the past, in the main for fellow doctors, but this short book is primarily addressed to the layperson. Many questions necessarily still remain unanswered: one man can only do so much and, as I said, I hope others will carry further this area of knowledge.

As a practising physician, I have always felt a sense of responsibility to those following my ideas and have always tried to be available not only to my patients through personal consultations, phone calls and letters but also to those reading my books. To this end, it was my practice to include my address and phone number at the end of all my books. Now that I am 90 years old, I feel that the time is approaching when I shall no longer be in a position to offer such on-going contact and advice. I am therefore writing this current book not with the aim of passing on details of the treatment of individual diseases – that can be found in my other books – but rather as a straightforward and, I hope, clear record of my observations and findings.

What I have to report is mostly favourable, my method frequently offering as it does not only considerable help to the sufferer but often the best hope of recovery. It can lead to profound changes for the good, but also for ill if used or initiated inappropriately. So in order to carry out my treatment safely and beneficially, there is a need for moderation and much common sense; there are also specific cautions to be observed and these I shall detail later.

I sincerely believe that both drugs and surgery should be used as infrequently as possible in the treatment of disease; however any discontinuation of medication or adjustment of dosage for those undertaking my method needs to be under medical guidance and the patient's progress carefully monitored. It is therefore imperative that patients with serious illness should place themselves under the care of a physician, if possible one experienced in the use of this method of treatment.

This book is not intended as a set of D-I-Y instructions* for the layman; I am well aware of the difficulties of following such a path on one's own. This being so, I include neither recipes nor the carbohydrate tables that were in some of my previous books. My aim is rather to tell my own story: namely, to write an accessible account of my medical work over time, including the lessons I learnt. I do this in order that others may avoid some of the pitfalls and derive some of the benefits of using this remarkable tool for treating illness non-invasively. I hope it will prove a useful resource for those interested in the subject, a contribution to the current debate on nutrition and health and a source of information for those wishing to try my method for themselves.

What I have to say is, I know, controversial. Yet so important is this way forward not only in the natural treatment of disease but also for overall health that I invite readers to come with me step by step on my journey of discovery, to share my thoughts and my findings and so to make sense of what I say for themselves.

My own beginnings

The story I am about to relate is also to some extent my own life story because, as well as with my work as a practising physician, my medical discoveries have also been intimately bound up with my own person. As I was already in my middle years when my new awareness came about, perhaps it is appropriate to first introduce myself by saying a little about my background.

Medicine was in my family. My father, Roman Lutz, the last child of a large family, was from the Tyrol and studied medicine at Innsbruck. The money his father had left him having more than run out, he moved to Upper Austria where he worked as a general practitioner. In 1912, after marrying my mother, the daughter of a classical scholar, my father opened a medical practice in Haag am Hausruck*, a village in the foothills of the Alps, Upper Austria. The local hospital was in Linz on the river Danube, and it was there that I, Wolfgang Joseph Theodor Lutz, was born on the 27 May 1913.

Physically, I was quite a puny child with underdeveloped muscles and so with poor posture. Nevertheless, I grew to have a love of outdoor sports, even if it was more love than aptitude! I spent four years at the Volkschule (primary school). Then, on the advice of my maternal grandfather, a high-ranking official, I attended for eight years the school attached to the Benedictine monastery of Kremsmünster, where, I remember, I did well. So you see, I made up for my poor physique by being bright at my studies!

My early years as the son of a country GP left a lasting impression on me, for sometimes in the school holidays I would accompany my father as he did his rounds to visit patients. It was a rural area with scattered homesteads and in wintertime we would both of us go on skis. I recall this so clearly. Many patients lived on outlying farms where there was little access to medical care and so, when my father called, he did whatever was necessary: treating his patients' ailments, even pulling their teeth and treating their animals!

These land folk had plenty to eat but even as a boy I noticed how ill they often were. I remember them having varicose veins and bad teeth, with no teeth left at all by the age of forty; they also had arthritis, cancer, strokes and so on. If only these people had known what I was to learn later, there might have been far less ill health amongst them – and that, of course, is why I am telling my story.

In his spare time, my father kept bees and, when I was in my teens, he was chairperson of the local beekeepers' association. I assisted him in this with some enthusiasm and gradually built up my own collection of hives. By the age of 23, I had sixty of them and was already researching and writing papers on bee-keeping.

Following in my father's footsteps, I read medicine. Like him, I studied at the Tyrolean University of Innsbruck, but also in Vienna. Again I passed my exams with flying colours. After graduating, I joined the staff at the Second University Hospital in Vienna, and immediately began scientific research there, as this was my foremost interest at that time. Internal medicine, too, was already beginning to fascinate me. During my time there, I did some work on the absorption of dyes and the entero-hepatic circulation (the circulatory link between the intestines and liver), publishing several papers on the subject*.

In particular, I worked on the intravenous injection of an iodine-containing compound, as iodine acted as a dye in the investigation of gallstones. During the inactive periods of digestion, the liver normally excretes bile to be stored in the gall bladder, ready for the next big meal. If iodine-containing X-ray contrast media is injected, the liver excretes this along with bile and a concentration of iodine builds up in the gall bladder and thus any gallstones present are highlighted under X-ray. It was known that, by injecting sugar in addition to the iodine, it would be possible to influence the transport of the iodine through the liver to the gall bladder in a way that would enhance the X-ray picture.

I felt that I was on the brink of a discovery in this transport system, but this was not to be: it was already 1937 and, by then, war was looming and the focus of my work had to change.

My paternal grandfather had been in commerce, trading between Austria and Italy. His father, that is my great-grandfather, came from Lake Constance and was a talented carpenter. He possessed much technical expertise, and had made his fortune by constructing a very successful automated watermill, powered by the river Ache on its way from the Achensee through the Tyrol. My great-grandfather was so proud of his constructional work that, in oil paintings of him, a drawing pad can always be seen at his side as well as a circle representing a mill wheel. My hope was that he had passed on his inventive streak to me and perhaps it was so.

As my heart lay in my scientific work, when war threatened I wondered if I could do something in this line to avoid being drafted. I therefore approached the German Luftwaffe as I was sure there would be scientific problems to work on. I had heard of a particular professor who wanted to found an institute to study the medical aspects of flying; this he did, north of Munich. In the end, I managed to arouse the professor's interest and was to work in his medical research institute throughout the war.

Here, I was engaged in studying the urgent problem presented by sudden drops in pressure during high flying. Right from the start, I was convinced that, by the end of the war, we would be flying in stratospheric conditions. The cabins of pilots in high-flying aircraft were already pressurised: the problem came if for any reason this mechanism failed. At 12,000 metres the pilot could take remedial action, but if the pressure cabin failed at a much higher altitude, it seemed that the pilot lost consciousness and fatalities ensued. Why was not known. The war industry was working on these high-flying jets and many people were trying to solve this in their own way, including fitness training for pilots. I remember, for example, one Prussian doctor thinking the pilots could be brought to withstand low oxygen pressure by high altitude training in the mountains, which was, of course, nonsense.

I myself felt that first it was necessary to understand exactly what was going on. I therefore devoted my attention to the transition reactions of warm-bloodied animals to a sudden drop in air pressure and built a little testing chamber to be connected to the big low-pressure chamber in which we used to investigate the reactions of pilots. My interest, of course, was in the reaction of humans, but I worked exclusively with South American rodents and rats, since I was convinced there was no difference in principle between the reaction of small warm-blooded animals and of larger ones like ourselves.

At the time, other flight researchers thought that the loss of consciousness suffered by pilots was because of the bubbles that arose in the arteries. However, as I studied the problem, it became clear that brain function was interrupted and consciousness lost at the actual moment in which the pressure dropped. I could see on the X-rays of the animals that it was only later that multiple bubbles arose in the arteries, and that these bubbles were caused by the difference in the pressure of the various gasses in the air at that height, differences which I simulated in my test chamber.

In other words, it was not the bubbles but the sudden drop in oxygen pressure that caused rapid loss of consciousness, rendering the pilot incapable of thinking and so allowing insufficient transition time for remedial action. Accordingly, I invented an airtight suit, which, when the oxygen pressure dropped below a certain amount, automatically inflated to a minimum pressure to prevent loss of brain function. It was a short-acting device, in principle like that still seen nowadays worn by astronauts working outside the space shuttle, only the oxygen flask was to be worn on the leg.

Anyway, this I designed, tested on my animals and wrote up in a report (Lutz 1942). By 1941 we were flying at 12,000 metres but certainly intended to fly at over 20,000 metres. Interest in this subject was therefore intense and my ideas reached the chief medical officer of the Luftwaffe in Berlin. I had worked only on animals, as I had always held human experimentation to be not only dangerous but also unnecessary and unethical. However, the prospect of this now arose and naturally I did not want to participate. Making various excuses, I managed to demur and the work was taken out of my hands and transferred to Berlin for further development.

I then moved on to the problem of saving the lives of pilots who had come down in Arctic waters. This meant working on various aspects of loss of body heat, including the very real possibility of the airmen freezing to death before rescue was possible when swimming in such icy conditions. Here again I worked on animals. I managed to show that warm-blooded animals needed not only warmth but also artificial respiration, since the brain woke later than the heart and there was therefore danger of suffocation. I was not a little proud when I managed to develop a technique to resuscitate warm-bloodied animals after more than 60 minutes of continuous cardiac arrest at a body temperature of about 0 degrees centigrade. I hoped too, that this technique might be useful for heart surgery and feel it could be useful today, for instance in avalanches.

In 1943, I was granted a postdoctoral degree in internal and flight medicine from the University of Vienna, in recognition of about 20 scientific papers that I had written both during my three years at the University Hospital and during the war. Austria had become part of Germany in 1938 and so the Austrian universities granted German qualifications. I therefore received the German distinction of 'Habilitation'* – hence the title 'Dr med. habil.' before my name, which I still carry. From the University of Vienna, I was also awarded the title 'Privat Dozent', an honorary lectureship, though this was never confirmed as, by then, the Russian army had taken Berlin; it was however honoured afterwards in Austria.

The war came to an end and I, like a great many others at the time, was put in prison, where I spent months. At this point, many German scientists were offered work abroad and so it was with me: I was offered a contract by the American military to work on the Apollo mission at the rocket centre of Wernher von Braun at Huntsville, Alabama. Perhaps I could have made a contribution there, I do not know. At the time, I did not want to go to America. My wish was to return to Austria – to go back to my family and to treat the sick in my own homeland.

I then spent two fairly uneventful years in camps. Sadly, air pressure experiments had indeed been carried out on human beings during the later part of the war and now the search was on for German doctors who had done these in concentration camps. As originator of suits for stratospheric decompression, the finger of suspicion understandably pointed at me. The idea for the space suits may have been mine, but I had not been involved in looking for proof on humans. Investigations showed that I was in no way connected with human experiments. My innocence being established, at the Nuremberg trials I was called only as a witness against those who had undertaken such despicable deeds.

In 1947, I returned to Haag am Hausruck, the village in Upper Austria where I grew up. Here, for a while, I joined my father's practice. Thus from being a medical scientist, I became a practising physician. A couple of years later I moved to the small town of Ried im Innkreis, also in Upper Austria, and here I opened my own practice in internal medicine*.

It was in Ried* that I was working, when, in 1957, I reached the age of forty-four: namely, the time when the story in this book really begins.

The puzzle of so much serious disease

As a young doctor leaving medical school, I had already been puzzled by the prevalence of so much serious disease. Even in those days, I had often wondered what it was that caused so much ill health. I had long felt that some factor in our civilisation must be responsible: such as the kind of life we led nowadays.

Perhaps the present level of physical activity was not high enough to sustain health? Yet I already knew that want of exercise was not the whole story, for these complaints were common amongst my father's and now my own farming patients who worked physically on the land from dawn to sundown. Was it because we cooked our food or that our food was too denatured in other ways? Or did the adding of salt do the damage? Amongst other things, the seemingly excessive intake of calories also concerned me, as did the eating of so-called junk foods – foods pleasurable but injurious.

I still regarded these factors as important but, the longer I worked with the sick, the more I felt there was something going on that was of even greater importance. I had now been in clinical practice for ten years and during this time I had seen a lot of serious medical conditions, especially the so-called 'diseases of civilisation' – conditions that medicine seemed to be at such a loss to prevent or to treat other than by drugs or surgery. By 'diseases of civilisation', I refer to those conditions often characterised by nutrient surplus and hence also called diseases of affluence: these include obesity, Type-II diabetes, heart infarcts, strokes, cancer, arthritis, gout, arteriosclerosis, certain intestinal ailments and dental caries.

As I write this book at the beginning of the twenty-first century, I am all too aware of the continuing increase in many of these complaints. When I started out in practice, morbus Crohn, for example, was a rarity and we hardly saw ulcerative colitis yet, over the next thirty years or so, I was to see and treat an ever-growing number of cases of both these debilitating bowel diseases.

My awareness of these ailments was also closer to home as I had witnessed much serious disease in my own family. True, I knew of no ulcerative colitis or Crohn's, but there were many instances of cancer and heart problems. Moreover, by now, my own health was in considerable trouble, so the puzzle had also become a personal one.

The state of my health by the mid-1950s

So here we are in the year 1957. I must dwell on this stage in my life story in some detail, as it has an important bearing on my future work as a doctor. I was approaching a turning point in my thinking both in regard to my personal health and in my approach to medical treatment.

By this time, as I said, my own health was in considerable trouble. An inflamed joint on my right index finger meant that I could not turn on a light switch, let alone perform the rectal palpations on my patients that my work as a doctor of internal medicine demanded. In fact, this intrusive arthritis at the end of my forefinger was the initial – and painful – spark, which kindled my awareness of just how far my health had already deviated from the ideal to which a man in his mid-forties fondly imagines he still conforms!

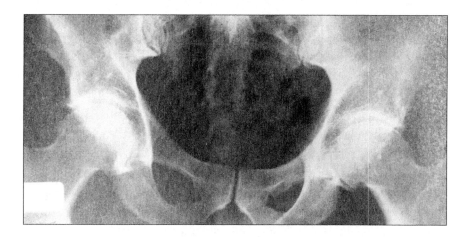

Figure 1.1: The hips of Dr Lutz showing osteoarthritic changes

Previously, though I had never been much of a sportsman, I had nevertheless really enjoyed sailing and skiing. Now I was seldom able to participate in such hobbies. For the last eight years, possibly more, I had been suffering from osteoarthritis of both hips. I walked with a limp, sometimes using a stick or umbrella for support. My shoes had been built up with soft rubber heels, but the pain in my hips was increasing steadily. My X-rays showed severe deformation of the joint surfaces of both hips, as those who can read X-rays can see in Figure 1.1. One day, I took them to show a colleague in Vienna. Thinking they were the X-ray pictures of one of my patients, he said: "Well, there's not much you can do for this case!" You can imagine the additional jolt this gave to my consciousness.

I was also liable to infections: enteritis in the summer and, in the winter, colds and coughs together with a recurrence of the herpes simplex virus, meaning weeks of unstable health following the period of fever. My skin was sensitive to pressure and easily chafed; my feet were subject to corns and my hairline was receding at an alarming rate. I know that my temperament was far from equable. I also felt driven and I was somehow anxious and always fearful of bad news.

But the worst of it was the devastating effect that my decline in health was having on my professional life. Because of the condition of my hips, sitting at an ordinary writing desk was scarcely possible. Minor incidents would lead to explosive outbursts of irritation. Moreover, since my youth, I had been plagued by migraines and had had to reckon with an attack even from running across a sunny playground during gymnastics. Recently, my migraines had been getting steadily worse, so that they, too, were now interfering with my work.

I have already mentioned my unserviceable forefinger. Added to this, overwhelming tiredness often kept me from working for more than two hours at a stretch and, after work, I would sometimes lie for hours, feeling totally exhausted. Yet this peculiar tiredness was combined with a sort of inner unrest, which prevented peaceful recuperation.

I had always been accustomed to the standard fare of any

reasonably well-off Austrian in the first part of the 20th century and had never paid much attention to what I ate. That being said, I had already noticed that this condition of unrest was provoked, or at least exacerbated, by meals containing a large amount of carbohydrate. At the time, I assumed this was to do with a sort of secondary adrenal insufficiency* for, though adrenal tests on me were normal, my restlessness certainly responded to cortisone. In the end, I was needing a cortisone preparation almost every day in order to continue in my professional capacity; very often I also needed a sleeping pill at night. So much for the state I was in at that time!

With the family background that I possessed, and with my own health so severely compromised, I feel that I very probably owe my life to what happened next. Be that as it may, I am quite sure that I owe to it the fact that, at ninety, I am busy working on my next article.

Turning point

It was during a holiday abroad I got an inkling of a possible answer to what had been puzzling me. Now, I have always loved fast cars and, in the mid-1950s, I had bought a new Citröen DS 19 in Paris. Wanting to go on holiday but being anxious about getting possible repairs to the car carried out well, I felt the safest thing to do was to holiday in or near France. Accordingly, I took my vacation in northern Spain and southern France. This was in 1957; the car has long since been traded in, but the influence of that memorable holiday is with me still.

Whilst on holiday, I had decided to make a tour of sites of Paleolithic art and it was in this way that I came to see the amazing cave paintings that were to set me thinking. After Spain, I had been to visit the prehistoric sites in southern France, including those of Les Eyzies, Lascaux and Trois-Frères. The colourful wall paintings in all these ancient caves greatly impressed me. There were wild horses, bison, musk oxen, cave bears, aurochs, shaggy ponies and reindeer, all so magnificently and so realistically portrayed. There were also larger animals such as the woolly rhinoceros, the elephant and the woolly mammoth. Were all these animals game animals, I wondered?

According to prehistorian Herbert Kühn*, the decorated parts of these caves, which often lay in very deep recesses underground, were not lived in; it was only the entrances that showed signs of human habitation. Rather they had an air of sacred mystery and probably served as some sort of ritualistic meeting place for Ice-Age hunters (Kühn 1954). The idea that the animal paintings had served some unknown magical purpose excited the medic in me and I pictured the hunters performing sacred rites before the hunt to propitiate the spirits of these wonderful animals. The paintings were so alive, so immediate. Perhaps it was this immediacy combined with the antiquity of the paintings that so sparked my imagination.

For spark my imagination they certainly did. I began to realise how much these ancient people must have relied on animals like these to provide them with the necessities of life – with skins and furs for their clothing, with bones for their tools (for instance, knives, needles and harpoons), with oil for their cooking and lighting, and above all to provide them with food. You see, these cave paintings are thought to date from the Paleolithic period and to have been drawn 30–13,000 years ago, so we are speaking of Europe during a very cold part of the last great Ice Age. Given the harsh climatic conditions at that time, their food must have consisted almost entirely of meat and meat fat. No wonder that so many pregnant females were depicted: it was vital that these animals flourished and reproduced, since on this the very lives of these nomadic hunters and their families depended.

The holiday had certainly been a stimulating one, but I had no idea at the time that my visit to the prehistoric caves was to set me off on a new track in my medical career. However, on my return home, I chanced to read an article in the *Journal of the American Medical Association* given by Dr George L. Thorpe from Wichita, Kansas; it was entitled 'Treating Overweight Patients'. Highlighted on the first page was an inset, which started:

> The simplest to prepare and most easily obtainable high-protein, high-fat, low-carbohydrate diet, and the one that will produce the most rapid loss of weight without hunger, weakness, lethargy, or constipation, is made up of meat, fat, and water.

I read on. It was good to read in the body of the article that:

> . . . a person can accomplish weight reduction without suffering slow starvation, prostrating weakness, agonising hunger pains, or the cynical remarks of friends . . .

Here was someone giving an address* to the American Medical Association who was talking of treating the obesity of his patients with a diet consisting mainly of protein, fat and water – in fact, a diet not dissimilar to that of the Ice-Age hunters whose caves I had just visited. (Note that even a diet consisting exclusively of animal food necessarily contains a small quantity of carbohydrate: glycogen, for instance, a type of animal starch found in muscle meat and liver.)

True, in practice Thorpe was using a slightly modified version of an Ice-Age diet, sometimes adding a little fruit and vegetables to avoid monotony, but I soon learnt there were other doctors in his circle in America, who were going almost the 'whole hog' as it were, at times putting overweight patients on a regime consisting purely of meat, with three parts lean to one part fat (by weight) and with the one concession to modernity of black coffee. The summary of Thorpe's article reads as follows:

> The patient with excess weight not caused by disease must be dealt with as an individual whose excess weight may be due to excessive carbohydrate intake or a disturbance of his carbohydrate metabolism. Evidence from widely different

sources . . . seems to justify the use of high-protein, high-fat, low-carbohydrate diets for successful loss of excess weight. There are apparent defects in the rationale of the commonly used low-calorie restrictive diets, and *there should be a return to a more natural type of diet*. Drugs may be used, but their defects should be considered. Common foods such as cereals and milk are excellent, but, in my way of thinking, they have no place in the diet of the overweight individual.

Thorpe (1957)

It was interesting that Thorpe thought cereals and milk unsuitable food for the obese. But what stayed in my mind – and the italics are mine – was Thorpe's phrase: 'a return to a more natural diet'. A short while later, an idea struck me; it was a flash of insight, if you like.

Crucial questions

My inspiration was to ask a crucial question: namely, if obesity had responded to 'a more natural diet' of mainly protein and fat, then might not other of our modern diseases do likewise? Why just obesity, why not high blood pressure, arteriosclerosis, cancer or gastrointestinal disorders? On the face of it, it was a most unlikely proposition. Yet, minor modifications apart, surely each nutrition-related condition couldn't require a different diet?

Once it had come to me, this challenging notion brought a great many questions in its wake. Was a diet mainly of protein and fat really a 'more natural diet', as Thorpe had suggested? Indeed, did we – did omnivorous Homo sapiens – have a 'natural diet'? In other words, was there a type of basic nutrition, specific to humankind as a species? I reasoned that animals of other species had a specific type of diet (at least in terms of its composition), so surely the same had to apply to humankind? If so, could it be that our Ice-Age diet was our natural one, for were not these people our own kind?

It was in searching for answers to some of these questions that evolutionary history provided me with a perspective on medicine, which has guided and sustained me to this day. Given the disarray in current nutritional thinking – disarray, which was already emerging in the late 1950s, it was interesting to discover a surprising level of agreement as to the dietetic history of evolving man. Indeed, it seems to be widely accepted still that man evolved as a meat-eater (by meat, I include any food of animal origin: insects, birds, eggs, shellfish, fish, small and large animals). If we include the meat-eating hominids, Homo erectus and archaic humans, this development took place over several million years. Biological anthropologist Rob Foley (1997) places the length of this evolutionary period as six to eight million years.

Thus, by the time we moderns came on the scene sometime between 100,000 and 200,000 years ago, the eating of meat as a staple food was firmly established in our predecessors, and also in our contemporaries for at this time the predominantly meat-eating Neanderthals were still roaming parts of the globe. Therefore, though this may not be a very palatable thought to some, it is nevertheless hardly surprising that we ourselves should arrive on the scene relying on animal food as our main source of nutrition.

There seems to be a general consensus that human beings emerged as a distinct anatomical species in southern Africa. When food got scarcer, some groups of Homo sapiens followed the game as far as South-east Asia and later up through the Middle East and on to Europe, where they are thought to have arrived some 30–40,000 years ago. Europe at that time was in the grip of the last Great Ice Age. The paintings in the prehistoric caves had been a powerful reminder of the fact that the first thoroughly modern humans to have arrived in Europe, the robust Cro-Magnon people in the Upper Paleolithic, were meat-eaters not only by descent, but also by environmental and climatic necessity.

To me, these small roaming bands of nomadic Cro-Magnon people were conveying a clear message: i.e. that having evolved to derive the vast majority of their calories from animal protein and fat, by continuing to live on animal food they were fit and strong enough to be able to withstand extreme cold; they were also courageous and clever enough to adapt to this harsh environment*. In fact, it is interesting to note that it was – and, I believe, still is – widely agreed amongst those writing about this period that a diet consisting either entirely or almost entirely of food from the animal kingdom constituted an excellent form of nutrition, which gave health, strength and stature* to these our forefathers.

Walking in the alpine meadows near my home in Austria, I have often been struck by the dearth of edible plants – edible by us, that is. During the many thousands of years of barrenness and extreme cold that constituted the last Ice Age, plant food would have been minimal and sometimes non-existent for those living at the edge of the European ice sheets. This was the time before settled communities and agriculture; fruit and vegetables as we know them today did not exist. The mosses and lichens found on the tundra and in the coniferous forests were no food for the human gut. However, fortunately for our survival, we modern humans could not only eat but could actually thrive on the animals that grazed these plants.

About this time – in terms of my own story, we are still in the late 1950s – I came across anthropologist and Arctic explorer Vilhjalmur Stefansson, whose work came to be very influential on my thinking. As regards the place in our diet of meat versus vegetation, Stefansson put it this way:

> During the period before agriculture, it is chiefly in the tropics, and not everywhere there, that men could, as some do at present, live like their anthropoid predecessors and cousins by digging roots and tubers, collecting shoots, bulbs, buds, fruits and nuts, and by catching a few small creatures. Outside the tropics pre-farming man was necessarily in the main a hunter; secondarily he was the gatherer of such animal foods as worms, grubs and insects (e.g. locusts),

shellfish and fish thrown up along the beach, stranded seals and whales. He scouted around, no doubt, and competed with the hyena and vulture for the bodies of animals that had died of illness, accident or old age.

This necessarily almost complete dependence of pre-agricultural man on animal food is not confined to the grasslands of the world, tropic, temperate or arctic; it applies nearly as much to some temperate zone and most arctic woodlands, even to many tropic forests. Carl Lumholtz reports, for instance, that when he was with the tropical forest dwelling natives of N. Australia they lived mainly on animal food, and never ate anything of vegetal nature if flesh foods were available.

So from the time when our ancestors ceased being ape-like gatherers of monkey-food down to the substantial growth of agriculture, mankind lived through one or several millions of years chiefly on the lean and fat of animals. The exception to this would be some groups which drifted back into sub-tropical and tropical forests of that humid type which enabled the chimpanzee and gorilla to remain anthropoid.

Stefansson (1946)

What Stefansson did not know when he wrote this, was that the food of both apes and monkeys turns out to be far more mixed than he realised, with meat forming a significant, if small, part of their diet (McGrew 1992).

From the perspective of our evolutionary history, there did seem to be a good case for seeing animal food as the basis of the original human diet, supplemented occasionally in some areas by plant food. As I pondered all this, I felt that the carbohydrate consumption of our Ice-Age European forefathers i.e. people with all the features and characteristics of people today, had to be limited to the little found in animal food and in the occasional wild plant. I will return to this epoch in our history in chapter 7.

What happened next, as the old gave way to the new – the Paleolithic to the Neolithic – was a far-reaching sea-change, both literally and figuratively: a change in sea levels, in our climate and also a fundamental change in our food base. With the gradual retreat of the ice, sea levels rose and there was a gradual warming up of the climate. Slowly, there was a regeneration of plant life as successive plant communities recolonised the ground exposed by receding glaciers. There was also a change in the fauna: fewer big game animals were available, some becoming extinct, and the reindeer went north to be replaced by red and roe deer and many smaller mammals. Apart from in the far North, in Europe the change was largely from migratory animals to ones that stayed mainly in the same locality.

I cannot do justice here to the myriad changes that happened during this transition period. What is especially important to my story is a certain change in flora, in particular the advent of cereals. Dr Jacob Bronowski, in his book *The Ascent of Man*, pinpoints a fundamental reason why cereals had not previously figured to any extent in the diet of humankind, namely that cereals as we know them did not then exist: they were merely wild grasses. It was only in the Neolithic Age that: 'the happy conjunction of natural and human events created agriculture', for there occurred: 'a strange and secret act of nature' (Bronowski 1979): namely the appearance of a hybrid wheat*, amenable to cultivation by man.

This was a big step in the life of man both culturally and dietetically for, together with the domestication of livestock, the emergence of hybrid cereals – for something similar happened to barley and other cereals – ushered in a new era. The possibility of rearing, growing and storing food meant the possibility of mixed farming, of the establishment of settled communities, of feeding more people on one spot. Culturally, it marked the end of prehistory and the beginning of what we call 'civilisation'; dietetically, it marked the end of the food of the nomad and the beginning of a 'life with bread'.

Slowly and in piecemeal fashion, the practice of mixed farming (livestock rearing plus the cultivation of cereals) spread from Asia Minor throughout the whole of Western Europe. Within the space of a few thousand years (less than 10,000 years and in some parts a lot less than this), cereals gradually became a staple food. Was the 'happy conjunction' that created cereal farming an unmitigated blessing, I wondered? For cereals grains were a new food, full of concentrated starch and therefore food to which the human digestive system was unaccustomed. An even more recent arrival to our dining tables was sugar, another source of concentrated carbohydrate. More recently still has been the availability of a plentiful supply of fresh fruit all year round. Moreover, extra sweetness is deliberately cultivated in fruit and vegetables and this, too, adds to the load of carbohydrate in our diet.

We humans are long used to eating animal food – and meat is still essentially meat, even if domesticated. I reasoned that the metabolism of humankind had evolved for efficient survival on animal food over a very long period of time and that, even without the long history of meat-eating of our predecessors, the last Great Ice Age of roughly 100,000 years, had itself lasted long enough for people to adapt completely to the food of the time. Thus, our whole metabolism had evolved to work smoothly and efficiently on a certain type of diet or at least a certain balance of constituents. This is the way it happens in nature.

Some plant food we could, of course, tolerate* and cereals have been a useful and even necessary resource during the vast changes that have taken place over these last 10,000 years or so. But had our bodies really had enough time to adapt sufficiently to these more recent starchy foods, I mused, and especially to the great quantity of carbohydrate often present in our diet today? If our constitutions were geared to one type of dietary composition and we then moved onto another very different one, might not this place a great strain on our internal organs? Might not disturbance result that if not immediately would eventually, and perhaps inevitably, lead to damage and subsequent illness? Could it be that the very extent of our departure from our original Ice-Age diet was a root cause of the sort of serious disease I had in mind?

In our zoos, once no longer on the diet of raw meat they had eaten in the wild, the big cats languished, yet regained their health and even managed to breed, despite captivity and a foreign climate, when their natural i.e. meat diet was restored. Were humans now languishing just as the big cats had done, not for want of raw meat as such, as even the predecessors of humankind had known fire for cooking, but for want of the animal food that was natural to us? Or, looked at a different way, was this languishing something to do with trying to cope with too much food of a new and perhaps unsuitable type?

I thought, too, of the trouble we are having with our domestic animals. Dogs and cats, both naturally carnivorous, are increasingly fed cereal and even vegetables. Amongst them, we are seeing a mushrooming of diseases we think of as human 'diseases of civilisation' – of cancer, obesity and diabetes. Was this pure coincidence? Cats with tooth decay, cows with mastitis, hens with osteoporosis, hens dying of heart attacks. The list is endless. Yet, in the wild on their accustomed food, these diseases rarely occurred – 'diseases of domestication' perhaps?

Be that as it may, the biggest and most challenging question of all was this: would returning to something akin to our original diet help restore people to health? It was in attempting to answer this question that I was to spend the rest of my working life.

2   MY OWN DIETARY EXPERIMENT

A return to our ancient diet?

The idea of returning to something approaching our ancient diet was an exciting one. Whether the basic solution to our modern diseases could really be that simple was not a question I could begin to answer at this stage. It had worked for Thorpe and his colleagues in regard to obesity. But as far as I then knew, such a diet had not yet been adequately put to the test as a wider medical treatment. Certainly, as a specialist in internal medicine, the thought of returning to a food that, if I was right, was better suited to the internal workings of our body particularly appealed to me.

In the late 1950s, I was discovering this way forward for myself. Since then I have come to value the contribution to this field that had already been made by Doctors Alfred Pennington, Blake Donaldson, Richard Mackarness and many others. In fact, it was from Mackarness in his slender book *Eat Fat and Grow Slim* (1956) that I soon learnt about the ideas of those who, already in the 19th century, were connecting the production of body fat with the eating of 'saccharine and farinaceous foods'. I instance throat surgeon Mr Harvey, who believed that sugar and starch were responsible for obesity, and who slimmed William Banting* by the exclusion of these foods, allowing freely of everything else. After making known the undoubted success of this measure, the rebuff both Banting and his doctor received from the medical profession of the time was perhaps prophetic? But, at that time, I was largely unaware of precedents of any sort and was full of the freshness of new inspiration.

In any experiment, you first need the initial idea; secondly, to test out this idea; lastly (to see if you are any the wiser for what you have done), there is a need to step back and assess the result of the trial. With me, the first step – the idea – was by then well established: namely that a dietary composition akin to that of our distant forbears might go a long way towards solving many of our health problems. Naturally, I was keen to know if my idea would work: it was now time to take the second step and to test the water.

Creating a modern version of our ancestral diet

Eager to put my idea into practice, I soon set about creating a diet that was as far as possible a modern equivalent to my idea of our ancestral one. I wanted to create a practical diet, which was well suited to everyday life and easy for my patients to follow. I myself am very partial to good food and so to make it appetising was part of my plan. In any case, the more appetising the food, the more likely it was that people would not only take to this way of eating but also to stick with it in the long term, should that prove essential to their health.

As to the contents of the diet, I wanted these to be available in ordinary shops and supermarkets. Obviously, to be feasible at all, the diet would have to use foods available today. Yet, at the same time, the contents of the diet had to reflect that of our ice-age ancestors – a tall order, you might say, considering that many if not most of our present day foods did not even exist in those days and most that did could no longer be procured!

My way over these undoubted hurdles was to concentrate on the different food constituents. As already discussed in the last chapter, a predominantly animal food diet with a few wild plants as extras necessarily contained mostly protein and fat. My plan therefore – and this is important – was to try to mimic our forefathers' diet in this regard. Any restriction of these food constituents, I felt, was therefore unlikely to be necessary: if these were our heritage, natural appetite could probably be relied on as a regulator.

Not so with carbohydrate! The main difference between the composition of foods then and now being precisely the dramatic rise in both the proportion of carbohydrate in our overall diet and in the actual quantity of carbohydrate consumed, I felt it was crucial to keep the level of carbohydrate to a minimum. With enough vigilance, I felt this to be possible with modern foods. These days, not all but most pre-packaged foods have the carbohydrate content written on the packet so it would be fairly easy to calculate a prescribed carbohydrate allowance for the day, even whilst browsing amongst the shelves of a supermarket. Naturally, many foods contain a mixture of protein, carbohydrate and fat and in varying amounts and this had to be taken into account.

Thus, in my task of reconstructing the diet of the Paleolithic hunter, I had decided it was constituents that mattered, and in particular the carbohydrate level. But how was I to go about choosing individual food items?

In his article, Thorpe reported that he found cereals and milk excellent for the non-obese, but I was not so sure. Dating from early farming in the Neolithic period as they did, both these foods were fairly recent. Not only that, but I felt that the carbohydrate content of cereals was definitely too high and, at this point in time, I was wary of including grain i.e. any cereal food at all. Milk contained a certain amount of sugar (present as milk sugar or lactose), but I figured that at least milk was of animal origin, so could be allowed as long as an eye was kept on the amount taken and its carbohydrate content was included in the daily reckoning.

Other than milk, I decided there should be free choice of most dairy products, especially of cream and full-fat cheeses. These were not only easy to buy but were to modern tastes very palatable sources of animal protein and fat. Eggs, too, I would include and all other foods that were strictly of animal origin, whether meat, fish, shellfish or poultry.

Red meat – both the lean and the naturally occurring fat – would be fine. Both had an exceedingly long pedigree and I had no hesitation in incorporating these in my regimen. I thought again of the large chamber called the Hall of the Bulls at Lascaux and of the hundreds of magnificent reindeer depicted there. I thought, too, of the wonderful physique attributed to those ancient hunters who lived on such game. These thoughts sustained me, imbuing me with the courage to proceed with my idea in a medical climate, which, despite the work of Pennington et al. in America, I did not expect to be immediately sympathetic.

I had no clear notion of what I expected to happen by introducing such a way of eating, i.e. what changes I expected to be brought about. I certainly did not anticipate the profound repercussions on the body's physiology, which were to be wrought by such a seemingly simple change of dietary emphasis. At the time, it was very much a case of 'try and see', which put me on the spot since, as a doctor, I did not like to try anything on my patients that I had not tried on myself.

In the circumstances, the only thing for it was to take courage and try the diet out on myself. Obviously I could not test the response to very many diseases on my own person. Nor was I obese (if anything I was too thin), so I did not expect to lose weight. Yet, as I have already related, my health was in a poor state – poor enough to spot any improvement, should it occur.

Moreover, my own self was the research material I had most readily to hand. It is, I know, frowned upon to place much weight on personal observations of this sort. Yet what is more convincing to the doubting scientist – or the doubting medic for that matter – than to observe the effects of something first-hand?

And so, in March 1958, my dietetic experiment began.

Trying out my idea of our ancient diet

Please remember what I said about wanting to make my 'new' diet as close as possible, not to the detailed content, but to the COMPOSITION OF THE DIET OF OUR ICE-AGE ANCESTORS IN TERMS OF PROTEIN, CARBOHYDRATE AND FAT. Mindful of this proviso and keen to get started, I launched straight into a diet extremely low in carbohydrate. By 'straight into', I mean literally from one day to the next.

I was sitting at lunch one day, when the last link in my chain of thought fell into place. I said: "Right, from now onwards, no more carbohydrate", which was my way of saying that I would give up cereal foods entirely from that moment. (I was actually resolved to eat in practice very little carbohydrate of any description, but as cereals are a predominantly carbohydrate food, I tended to refer to them as 'carbohydrates'. It was my own short-hand, if you like.) This was just before leaving for a holiday in the Mediterranean.

With the wisdom of hindsight, I can see that my impulsiveness was not very sensible. I know a lot more now than I did then and if I were to repeat the experiment, I think I would start a lot more gradually. Be that as it may, I am telling of how I, myself, actually started 'living without bread': that is living with minimal carbohydrate in my diet. Without more ado, I cut right down on foods such as sugar, cakes, puddings, chocolate, fruit and potatoes, intending as I said to eat no bread or cereal foods at all. Beer somehow did not count.

This went well while I was still at home, as I could avoid dishes that were enticing but unsuitable by not having them on the table. Once on holiday aboard a passenger steamer, it was not so easy, for here I was constantly faced with a wonderful selection of mouth-watering Viennese pastries – a temptation to which, I must admit, I succumbed. After that holiday, I fared a lot better and managed to stick to the diet more or less the whole time.

Personally speaking, I took to my new diet very easily and did not find it much of a problem. I already ate meat and fats like butter and cream had long been a real pleasure to me. Traditional Austrian cooking is rich in animal fat, so I suppose I did not have the problem of habituating myself to what some might have found richer food than they were used to.

Gradually, I weaned myself from some of the foods to which I had been formerly accustomed. It was interesting how, little by little, I became indifferent to starchy foods. I hardly noticed the absence of 'fillers' like potatoes and pasta or bread. Eventually, I scarcely regarded them as food anymore. Admittedly, it was odd having no bread round my sandwiches and it felt a bit strange to my tongue the first time I tried a snack of just cheese with butter on, but I soon got used to it and even came to enjoy such a delicacy. However, sugar and sweet foods never lost their attraction for me and I got used to satisfying my 'sweet tooth' with small amounts of fruit or the occasional dessert such as ice cream or compote.

From then onward, animal food was the mainstay of my diet and, for about four years, I ate meat, meat fat, eggs and full-fat dairy produce, together with a few vegetable dishes and, now and then, a little fruit. I reckon the carbohydrate content of my experimental diet to have been about 20–30g per day. Strictly-speaking it must have been a little more than this, as I did not include carbohydrate from alcoholic drinks such as beer and wine, feeling that moderate amounts of alcohol (which is metabolised differently and which I now tolerated better) would do me no harm as long as I watched my other carbohydrates carefully enough.

To give the reader an idea of what I ate during those first experimental years, I include Figure 2.1, which offers a sample menu. Obviously, what I ate varied depending, for instance, upon whether or not we had guests, but given here is a fairly typical day's food for that time.

Breakfast: 1/2 pint of milk or 1/4 pint cream, with a raw egg
Coffee, black without sugar

Lunch: Mushroom or asparagus soup (made without flour), sometimes with the addition of egg or bone marrow.
Meat, preferably fatty, with salad or vegetables (French-style: with butter, no flour)
Dessert: Fruit salad, or a dish made from fresh white cheese, served with jam or stewed fruit (only slightly sweetened)
Alternatively, cheese with butter, or ice cream.
Coffee with cream

Supper: Cold cuts of meat, or hot meat again not too lean, occasionally with vegetables but without bread
Bottle of beer

Figure 2.1: A typical day's menu over these four years

Please note that this version of my 'pre-Neolithic' diet is fairly extreme and I DO NOT ADVOCATE STARTING A LOW CARBOHYDRATE DIET THIS WAY.

The above sample menu is therefore not at all prescriptive. There was very little carbohydrate in it. The dessert I chose to include served, it is true, as a comforting reminder of past culinary delights but I took only a very modest portion. After the first four years, I myself eased up somewhat and increased my amount of carbohydrate. As I gained more experience of the diet, I found that a more moderate version worked perfectly well.

The above is therefore not illustrative of the diet I came to use on a regular basis with my patients, which was to be slightly higher in carbohydrate and more liberal as to which carbohydrates might be included. In chapters 4 and 5, I will describe at some length my basic long-term regime and its implementation.

An evaluation of my four-year trial

So how did I feel on my new diet and what changes did I notice in myself? Well, I am pleased to report that, despite saying I would have done it differently nowadays, the changeover actually went very smoothly. In fact, even in the early days of my four-year trial, I noticed in myself such marked changes for the better that I soon became convinced that I was on the right lines.

At first, I was quite tired and obliged to go to bed early, but for that I awoke brighter the next morning. Indeed, as far as my work went, I was pleasantly surprised to find that, after only a few weeks, I could start doing more than previously in my practice. Gradually, I gained in stamina and was able to work more quickly and to accomplish my work in better humour. The pain in my forefinger eased after a few months. My decision-making speeded up, as did the time it took me to do dictations and X-ray examinations. Eventually, I coped with the demands of full-time work without tiring – and have been working hard ever since!

My mental state, too, underwent a change. I became calmer and got more joy from life. I lost the feeling of constant inner restlessness as well as the sense of foreboding that had plagued me. In fact, I have the impression that I became a more balanced person – but my colleagues and family are perhaps better judges of that! One thing I found, and which I only really noticed in retrospect, was how much better I was reacting in dangerous situations. No longer did my heart thud in traffic, for example, and no longer did I panic and break out in a sweat when things were stressful: now I stayed calmer and I only sweated when my temperature needed regulating, and then I perspired profusely and not at all unpleasantly.

A noticeable improvement also took place in the quality of my skin. It became stronger, was less liable to fungal attack and became able to withstand hours of manual work without trouble.

Corns became a thing of the past and even that appendage of skin, my hair, had its share in the benefits. It soon became obvious that my scalp was in far better condition than it had been and that my hair had stopped falling out. Of course, I had hoped that the bare patches would be 'reforested', but at least the 'forest boundaries' have been maintained.

Something else, too, I noticed about my skin was a change in oiliness. Right at the beginning of the change of diet, my skin became very dry as though its lubrication had dried up. Then, later, a different and oilier type of fat made its appearance on my skin, more like that described as characteristic of the skin fat of various peoples still living in the wild. Perhaps the retreat of acne on this diet is linked to such changes? By and large the production of firm earwax was lessened, a change clearly visible on a doctor's instruments.

Progress with my migraines was not straightforward. Initially, I quickly became almost free of attacks. But after about six months of the diet, my migraines returned and actually got worse, which I probably brought upon myself. Delighted that I could now tolerate coffee so much better and without any accompanying nervous excitation, I had begun to drink more and more of it! Once I moderated my coffee habit and had taken up sport again, my migraines assumed bearable proportions, which I could control with the usual tablets. After a while, I ceased to need medication and eventually said a grateful good-bye to migraines altogether.

During my four-year trial, my dental health also improved. Before my change of diet I had needed dental repair work for caries every six months, yet dental caries, like corns, now became a thing of the past. I felt good in myself, slept better than before and, moreover, experienced a steady and enduring improvement in my digestion. I must also mention the fact that I had noticeably fewer infections than formerly and, if I did have one, I was far less inconvenienced by it.

Remember I used to experience frequent and sometimes excrutiating exacerbations of the arthritis in my hips, so you can imagine my delight when, after about six months on the diet, my hip pains began to lessen. After eight or nine months my hips improved considerably. These flare-ups disappeared, as did the morning aches and pains across my sacrum, and I no longer limped. In fact, my arthritic pains gradually seemed to melt away and my hip joints now only made themselves felt during an infection or when I twisted suddenly or too far.

I had long since abandoned skiing because of my hips and also because of my former constant tiredness and consequent lack of interest in physical activity. On the diet, not only had the symptoms of my arthritis lessened but also my muscles were increasing in strength, as were my powers of endurance. I needed these various improvements to enable me to return to sporting activity and I was pleased indeed when I found that I was able to begin to do a little skiing with my children. Later I was to take up tennis again.

The reader will be wondering about my weight during this time. Well, I had been too lean before the change of diet and had weighed only 65kg. I lost 1½ kg at first, about which I was none too satisfied, but which I put down to a mobilisation of fat reserves as well as a loss of water. After a few months my weight loss ceased and, from then on, my weight rose slowly and steadily. I am 176 cm tall and, by the end of four years of carbohydrate restriction, I weighed a good 79kg and I like to think I looked better for it! I certainly felt it.

I had lost the pain in my forefinger, as I said, after a few months on the new food regime. What I then noticed was that my fingers and wrists were becoming sturdier. Gradually I found that I could not wear my old rings anymore, yet my fingers were by no means fat, just more substantial. Likewise, though I had gained about 14kg in total bodyweight, my layer of body fat had not seemed to alter to any great extent. I therefore ascribed both my new ring size and my weight gain to an increase in body mass rather than of fat.

Indeed, this increase in body mass, i.e. in skin, bone, connective tissue and muscle bulk is an interesting phenomenon, which seems to happen automatically on a low carbohydrate diet – even without any increased physical activity on the part of the person concerned. Here was I, a doctor of nearly fifty years of age, with far fewer possibilities to do physical training and yet with a stature more impressive than I had possessed as a medical student 30 years before!

In fact, I felt so well that I took little heed of the well-meaning questions from family and friends: "Are you not afraid to pursue a diet, which is in stark opposition to the opinions of the universities and which you yourself have only cursorily checked out?" No, I was not afraid. However, I was eventually persuaded by apprehensive colleagues to check my cholesterol level – a thing to which I attached little importance at the time. So, thanks to Dr Leopold of the University Hospital of Cologne, after three years of eating plenty of animal fats, my blood lipids were measured. They were all found to be low. (For your interest, I give the results in chapter 8, Figure 8. I.) At the time, I also had other tests such as urine tests, tests for uric acid, GOT, Rest-N, morphological blood findings, an electrocardiogram and so on: all showed normal values. After this, I was not much concerned about my cholesterol or other levels.

I wrote up my report of my personal dietary trial in 1962, in an article entitled 'Vier Jahre ohne Kohlenhydrate' (four years without carbohydrate) in *Medizin und Ernährung* (medicine and nutrition). Over the years, by writing up my observations and findings as I went along, I compiled a sort of diary, a chronological record of my journey of discovery. This I did, first in articles and later in books. There is a list of my publications* at the end of this book.

Naturally, starting the diet at 45 years of age in such poor health, and with osteoarthritic changes already well established in my hips, there were bound to be limits as to what a diet could achieve. Yet, even if the diet did not solve all my health problems, I was still pleased with its effect on me. So much so that, with my increased competence at work and the tendency for me to be in a better mood, I could not now think of returning to what I used to consider as 'normal' food.

3 EARLY WORK WITH PATIENTS

Previous experience

My own trial was my first personal experience of partaking of a low carbohydrate diet, but it was not in fact the first time I had come across one. I had already met low carbohydrate nutrition in a clinical setting when I was working in Vienna at the Second University Hospital after qualifying as a doctor. There, I used to visit a colleague who worked in the outpatient clinic for diabetics, and so had the opportunity to observe the results of the treatment of individual patients. This was in the 1930s before the routine clinical use of either insulin or oral antidiabetics.

The good outcomes achieved by this clinic were noteworthy. It was here that I had learnt that straightforward cases of what we then called adult-onset diabetes – and now call Type-II diabetes as it is no longer confined mostly to old age but tends to happen earlier and earlier – responded very well to a low carbohydrate diet. This was something I was soon to rediscover in my own medical work. Moreover, the clinic diet was very successful in preventing many of the degenerative changes that have come to be expected as an almost inevitable part of the disease. This avoidance of the unfortunate and distressing 'side effects' of diabetes through dietary treatment I was also to witness in my own later work. Oh, how much suffering could be averted if this were better known!

The dietetic regime then in use was that developed by Professor Carl von Noorden* before the First World War. It provided ample protein and offered fat as a better general energy source than carbohydrate; if necessary, patients were encouraged to add fat to their food: to do so was not seen as a problem in those days. This regime was not quite as low in carbohydrate as mine had been during my four experimental years, but very low by today's standards. Importantly, the diet restricted carbohydrate sufficiently to stabilise the blood sugar of many of the patients that came to the clinic with diabetes.

To all intents and purposes, the diet used in that pre-war clinic conformed to my new conception of a 'Paleolithic' diet. However, in those far-off days, I saw a low carbohydrate diet purely as a part of the treatment for late-onset diabetes. Personally, I had not made any wider connections. It was only now – some twenty years later – that I began to realise that such a diet might be more widely applicable.

General benefits

A doctor's job is always to offer to his patients the best therapy he is able to. By the time I started my own personal dietary experiment in March 1958, I had already built up a fair-size practice specialising in internal medicine, and I now wished to put my new tool to therapeutic use. Here I must confess, so astounded was I by the rapid improvements shown on my own person, that I did not await the outcome of my four-year trial before doing so.

It was therefore not long before I was suggesting to some of my patients that they try the diet and, over the next few years, I was to advise many patients to cut down their carbohydrate intake, either to the minimal amount I was having myself in those early days or to the slightly higher amount that we had used at the diabetic clinic before the war.

The patients who embraced my dietary approach were suffering from a whole variety of disorders, but their reports of the general benefits that they derived from the diet had a lot in common. Today, I still receive letters asking about procedure in relation to a specific medical condition, which mention at the same time some unexpected but pleasing improvement in other seemingly unrelated aspects of the patients' health. The following excerpt is a recent example.

> I read with interest your brochure on low carbohydrate nutrition. For a few months now, I have been following your principles with great success. I have lost weight, my stomach is no longer so overacidic and my arthritic fingers hurt less.
>
> R X, Oxford

This was from a letter consulting me about a very different medical issue than the points mentioned. (I received this letter after I had issued an English synopsis of my main book in 1998.)

Many people told me I could use their names for this book and I thank them for this display of confidence in the diet. However, out of general discretion, I have changed the initials of every patient I mention. It goes without saying that the positive comments I received were very encouraging for me, since I was pursuing what was, medically speaking, quite a solitary pioneering path.

Let us take a look at some more of the 'unexpected but pleasing' general improvements, which were reported to me:

- Warmer hands and feet. Having cold hands and feet can be a misery. Yet, soon after starting the diet, many patients reported having warm hands and feet, sometimes for the first time that they could remember. I was to hear this time and time again. To me this indicated the improved circulation that I was so often to witness in my patients.

- Better skin. Some reported the disappearance of calluses and corns on their feet. Others found, as I had done, that the skin on their hands became tougher and chafed less easily, yet nevertheless was smooth and flexible. Still others were delighted by the disappearance of facial acne or by the emergence of a clearer facial complexion generally.

- Pleasanter sweat. Perhaps I might add that, on their new diet, the sweat of some patients became pleasanter and they experienced an absence of what is commonly called body odour: no longer did their clothes become discoloured at the armpits and the need for deodorants became a thing of the past.

- Better sleep patterns. Patients slept better, suffered less from bad dreams and woke more refreshed than previously.

- Less stress. Higher stress tolerance was noted. Some said that their partners found them easier to live with and felt that they were developing a more unruffled disposition since going on the diet; others noticed an increase in mental efficiency. All this suggested a beneficial effect on the nervous system. Certainly, I had soon discovered myself that a 'life without bread' had a most agreeably soothing effect on my nerves.

- Less overeating. A generally experienced benefit was the lessening of overall food intake: most patients felt less need to eat so much, less need to eat so often and actually ate a lot less in total quantity than they used to. The absence of incessant hunger was in itself a blessing for many: for people accustomed to an urgent need to eat every couple of hours, it was relaxing to be able to forget about food for hours at a time.

- Better digestion. Not only did people eat less by choice, but what they did eat, they seemed to digest a lot better, without any of the symptoms such as excessive wind or heartburn that had been previously troublesome. The diet, they said, was very undemanding on the stomach and gut. Lack of the stuffed-up, bloated feeling that meals had frequently engendered in the past, together with the disappearance of sleepiness after meals, was often commented on. These feelings of unaccustomed lightness and well-being all pointed to a new and most welcome digestive harmony.

- Easier bowel action. Those suffering from what we might call 'intestinal hurry' found more peaceful action with no need to rush. Others, who had been constipated, sometimes after initial trouble in adjusting, found bowel action became more regular. Flatulence was lessened; indeed, many patients were relieved to find that any wind they did pass was passed not only very easily but with no accompanying offensive smell, as were their motions, which over time became almost odourless.

- More energy. At first, some people felt the need to get more sleep, but this soon gave way to higher general energy levels and to the ability to work longer than before without fatigue.

- Better posture. Furthermore, many men were happy to report stronger, firmer muscles and improved physique – and this irrespective of the amount of exercise they did, as had happened with me. Women patients, too, gained stronger muscles, yet without any accompanying masculinisation and observed their new figures and better posture with contentment. Patients of both sexes slouched less, stood taller and sat up straighter than they used to without thinking about it and with more ease.

- Fewer infections. Another benefit frequently mentioned is that of seemingly increased resistance to infection: a remarkable number of patients commented on a lessening of the incidence of colds, influenza and infections generally. Later I was to learn something of the physiological mechanisms behind this improved resistance to infections, as we shall see later on.

- Female patients reported considerable benefits from

carbohydrate restriction in the sphere of reproductive health: menstruation was said to regularise and pregnancies to run smoothly, with no loss of figure after the birth. I remember in particular one young woman on my diet telling me of the ease and simplicity with which she gave birth – something not too common these days. For some of my women patients, even the menopause became the natural and untroublesome happening that surely nature intended it to be.

- Male patients also found differences. A university professor interested in diet once told me that he had tried reducing carbohydrate but that, even though he had felt exceptionally well and could work much more than usual, he had given it up again because his sexual potency had taken such a downward turn. Had I known at the time, I could have reassured him by forecasting that this initial loss of libido would right itself after a few months. Then, together with a disappearance of post-coital tristesse, there might well come an increase in potency, yet without the previous sense of being at the mercy of one's sex drive – no more being driven, rather being in the driving seat, as it were.

- Lastly, in old age, some reported feeling a second flush of youthful buoyancy, so perhaps my diet was even exerting a beneficial effect on the ageing process?

This was some of the positive feedback from my patients once I introduced carbohydrate restriction into my clinical work, many of these improvements becoming obvious to them very soon after trying the diet. Note: I cannot yet speak of 'my diet', for I had not yet settled on what that was to mean in terms of a daily quota of carbohydrate. Such benefits were still reported when I adopted a slightly higher quota and have continued to be reported ever since.

Several different improvements might occur simultaneously and, as I mentioned earlier, were not confined to the particular disease a patient had consulted me about: for instance, a patient with a bowel problem might report how his or her hands and feet were now warmer, or someone with an ulcer might report how much sounder they were sleeping or that their corns had vanished and so on. Moreover, the subjective reports of benefits tended to reflect fairly accurately the changes that, as a doctor, I witnessed in my patients and which I could measure and so verify objectively. It was rewarding feedback.

The slimming of young children

Given that it had been partly Thorpe's treatment of obesity that had initially prompted me to wonder about the wider application of carbohydrate restriction, it is hardly surprising that obesity was one of the first medical conditions to which I turned my own attention. (I am speaking here of treatment for the common type of obesity, not of the obesity that accompanies specific diseases such as Fröhlich's syndrome or hypothalamic obesity.)

In cities, childhood obesity fell within the province of the paediatrician, but working in a rural practice, as I did in those days, I saw many fat children. The parents who brought these young children to me – and here I am talking about children of either sex before puberty – were perplexed on two counts: firstly, they had been advised by their doctors to give their children less to eat and yet they found that the children themselves were often ravenously hungry and were in no mood to cut down on their food intake; secondly, they were to encourage their children to do sport and yet their children were too tired and unfit to enjoy taking up sport.

Overweight parents bringing overweight children would wonder if their children's obesity was hereditary, and, to some extent, this is probably so: certainly one sees families in which most of the members tend to overweight and later to diabetes. But having a predisposition towards a particular medical condition does not mean you necessarily have to either develop that condition or to continue to suffer from it, especially given due precautions. So I would say to the parents that, whether or not they (or the child's grandparents) were overweight, the child in question still had a chance of recovery: that we should give the diet a try and see if it did the trick.

Another question parents would frequently ask was whether they had been overfeeding their children. In answer, I would explain that it was **WHAT THEIR CHILDREN ATE THAT MATTERED RATHER THAN HOW MUCH** they ate. To be allowed to take as much as they liked of the allowed foods, could be a relief to the child who was used to quite a quantity of food on its plate. (That appetite tends to be self-limiting on this diet was something that a child would, in time, discover without any effort on his or her part.)

It was particularly necessary to reassure parents that their children would be well nourished and not suffer from any nutritional deficiency by eating this way. The belief in the necessity of eating carbohydrate-containing foods is deeply rooted in our culture, especially the need for good 'daily bread' and for fruit and vegetables as essential sources of vitamins – issues I will come back to in due course. Sugary soft drinks and fizzy drinks, seen by some parents as healthy for children, were to be totally avoided, as was even fruit juice.

I also found it necessary to protect adipose children as much as I could from the attentions of well-meaning grandmothers and aunts, who were so fond of handing these 'poor darlings' sweets and chocolates on the quiet. School breaks were another danger to the success of the attempt: if children were given cereal-free sausages or hard-boiled eggs for their snack, it was important that these were not swapped at playtime for buns, sweets or cake! A word in the ear of the teacher could be of great help here.

I would further reassure parents that the diet would restore both energy and good physique to their tired offspring – that, as long as they left the fat on the steak, the diet was, after all, similar to the 'steak and salad' diet popular at the time for athletes in training. (For I had noticed how, once on the diet, the posture of these children improved, how they became more upright, their swaybacks and even their knock-knees straightened out.)

With both parents and children, I would discuss the diet in detail. I would tell them that my young patients were allowed any amount of animal food they chose to eat (with the exception of milk, which was limited to a maximum of a pint a day); that they could also have a moderate amount of leafy or root vegetables (sautéed in fat, but without flour), as well as eating some green salad, tomatoes and mushrooms. All other foods were forbidden.

Notice that at first the children were not allowed any fruit, nor could they indulge in sugar or anything containing sugar, nor even any bread. The diet I was using at the time was very strict. However, though at the beginning they had to do without toast for breakfast, they could if they wished have egg and bacon and, though no chips, they could have sausages (100% meat) and tomatoes for lunch, and salmon steak and salad for tea. It was not such a bad prospect!

I would explain to parents, as simply as I could, that the carbohydrate we eat (sugar or starch) is converted in the body to sugar, which enters the bloodstream; that we do need a certain amount of sugar in our bloodstream, but that too much (or too little) is dangerous for health; that consequently, if a lot of sugar enters the bloodstream, the hormone insulin will take immediate action to remove most of it (i.e. bring the blood sugar down to a safe level), one of its ways – and the important one for the obese – being to convert the sugar to fat. Hence eating a lot of carbohydrate can mean a lot of insulin being produced by the body, which can soon mean a lot of stored fat!

This I told parents, because I found that their obese children were usually suffering from a condition known as hyperinsulinism. In other words, not only did they eat too much starchy and sugary food in the first place but also, in response to all those carbohydrates, their bodies secreted an excessive amount of insulin (more than needed to deal to with the resultant sugar), a phenomenon easily confirmed and, in time, usually amenable to treatment by a low carbohydrate diet. I also explained how this condition had been the reason for both the lethargy of their offspring (energy was used in creating fat) and their sometimes seemingly insatiable desire for food*.

When the goal had been achieved and the obesity conquered or under control, the forbidden foods were gradually reintroduced but strictly rationed. It was, of course, no good for the children to then return to their old ways. To stay slim, it was necessary for the children to stay on a level of carbohydrate that would not elicit a return of their hyperinsulinism: a level of carbohydrate I would clinically determine for the individual child by means of a glucose tolerance test, so that both parents and children knew exactly how to proceed.

In fact, the procedure I used then was very much like that subsequently used by Dr Robert Atkins (1972) in the treatment of obesity i.e. first to reduce carbohydrate to a minimum and then to monitor the effect of restoring carbohydrates to the diet in order to determine a suitable maintenance level, only for me the important level to monitor was not so much weight as the performance of the child's blood sugar.

With children, I found it wise not to watch the scales too closely: these children were still growing and so, as girth gave way to height during growth spurts, fat was replaced by noticeably improved muscle, connective tissue and bone (all heavier than fat). Consequently, whilst not necessarily lighter, the children grew slimmer and at the same time more robust. Sooner or later, the children would attain their ideal figure, by which I mean ideal for them, not a gaunt and over-thin product of fashion. Always remember that, yes, our human body is meant to be athletic, but not excessively skinny and this holds as true for children as it does for adults.

How long did it take? Except in very extreme cases, those children that persevered with the diet took at the most one year to look slim and healthy; more often than not, the process was completed within six months.

Young children, it seemed, adapted very quickly to a change in diet. As long as their health was not already too impaired, I found that they could be placed on a diet, even one ultra-low in carbohydrate, without delay. Here, it seemed to me, was a straightforward case of cause and effect: too much carbohydrate = too much insulin = too much body fat. Of course, I could only show this in reverse, i.e. that withdrawing the carbohydrate removed the body fat, and hence dealt with the obesity.

During my time in Ried, I treated over a hundred cases of childhood obesity. It is seldom one can claim so much, but I can happily report that, with young, pre-pubertal children, the success rate was quite astonishing. Without any calorie restriction whatsoever – as long as they stuck to the diet – as regularly as clockwork, every single obese child that I treated regained his or her slender figure. This ten-out-of-ten result was very gratifying.

The slimming of adults

These were early days in my dietary adventures – very much experimental days – and it is the lessons that I learnt during this time, which led me to formulate my own 'Plimsoll line' for therapeutic levels of dietary carbohydrate.

If the first lesson I learnt had been the quick adaptability of the very young, the second lesson was that this process was less straightforward when it came to treating adults: success was more variable and other factors seemed to enter the picture.

For these first few years working with the adult adipose – a kinder word than fat – I again used a diet that was extremely low in carbohydrate: namely, something like 12–20g daily. I allowed dairy produce and, to save greater temptation, the occasional indulgence such as a tiny amount of fruit compote or a very small portion of ice cream, just like I permitted to myself. These adults were self-monitoring and so I was not sure just how much carbohydrate they were actually eating, I think sometimes nearer 60–70g daily, but certainly a lot less than previously.

Weight loss was generally neither spectacular nor fast – which I would not in any case recommend, since it is far easier (and also far safer) for the body to accommodate itself to a gradual reduction in weight. But weight loss was usually steady and persistent and, provided that the patient stuck to the diet, the process would often continue unchanged for as long as it took to reach a steady weight. Adults generally lost about 3–4kg in the first month, about 2kg in the second month and thereafter roughly 1kg a month. In certain cases where overweight was either excessive or persisted despite the diet, I found it necessary not only to keep an eye on alcohol intake but also to restrict calories as well as restricting carbohydrate. In general, it was quite unnecessary to restrict or even count calories*.

With adults, too, I soon learnt not to confuse obesity with weight loss per se. Some people lost weight consistently, others even gained a little, especially at first. Still others lost weight so far and then remained on a plateau, and the higher the previous weight, the higher the plateau. As with children, it seemed that weight loss was partially counteracted by some extent of weight gain. This I put down, firstly to the marked improvement in tissue quality that tends to happen with carbohydrate reduction and, secondly to the maintenance of the normal layer of fat under the skin, which nature intended as a reserve for hard times – both probably due to a healthier level of growth hormone.

People therefore tended to become stronger, sturdier and more shapely. So, although a better, trimmer and pleasing figure was usually attainable for both men and women, those of mature years did not always lose as much weight as they wished. I know this could be a little disappointing for some patients who had sacrificed a lot of their comfort foods in the hope of gaining a really svelte figure. Looking back, I think one of the reasons my success with slimming adults was not quite the overwhelming success I had hoped for, is that most of my patients came from rural farming stock and tended to participate in communal meals, which rendered abstention or special catering more difficult. However, when they managed to follow it, patients usually felt well on the diet and, in many cases, were very happy with the results.

Incidentally, I found a low carbohydrate diet also advantageous to the over-thin, adults and children alike. (Remember I had been over-thin myself.) Gauntness is removed by the acquisition of a normal layer of subcutaneous fat, as one part of a whole change for the better: namely, the underweight seemed to profit from the same gain in body bulk (as opposed to excess body fat), which I was seeing in formerly obese patients. Thus, just as with flabby muscle that had run to fat, so, too, in the thin, did poor muscle that had been too puny regain its tone – again the action of the growth hormone?

Of course, I wanted the diet to work like magic, but conditions that have been present for, say, half a lifetime do not disappear overnight. I pondered why, when it comes to giving up fatty tissue, some people responded more readily than others to carbohydrate restriction. In both men and women, the already existing pattern of fat distribution seemed to influence progress (the pear-shaped in both men and women being the most reluctant to slim), as did the approach of the menopause in women (suggesting matters were being complicated by hormonal changes). The expanding of individual fat cells as opposed to the multiplication of fat cells also seemed to be an influential factor. Or could it be that some of the changes, which seemed to accompany obesity, persisted even though the nutritional cause of the obesity had now been removed?

Nevertheless, in the treatment of obesity, I thought it always worth trying the diet before resorting to harsher and more invasive methods, since I found that not only did most overweight people of either sex lose some weight when carbohydrates were limited, but I also felt that total bodyweight per se lost some of its significance as a risk factor given THE IMPROVEMENT IN OVERALL HEALTH, which I witnessed in these patients,

'It's my glands!'

The 'glands' were a popular focus of blame for obesity and many a parent would ask whether it was the 'glands' of their overweight teenager that caused the problem. Certainly, the glands were involved, especially the endocrine glands, but was it right to blame the glands themselves? I had already shown the link between high carbohydrate intake, the pancreas (and its hormonal messenger insulin) and obesity, and had pondered the probable role of the growth hormone (released by the pituitary gland) in reducing or enhancing tissue quality. Now other links were beginning to suggest themselves.

The feedback I was getting from adult patients who had cutback their carbohydrate intake significantly gave me one clue to follow up, for talk of more regular menstruation and easier childbirth, together with tales of a calmer and more fulfilling sex life indicated that restriction of carbohydrates might be having a beneficial effect on the sex hormone levels of my patients. However, these were necessarily subjective reports: objective assessment was necessary and sex hormones therefore became a focus of mine quite early on.

Together with Viennese endocrinologist Dr H. Iselstöger, I did some research. We started by looking at the sex hormone levels of obese adult patients eating their customary food and what we found was that these patients – of both sexes – showed raised levels of oestrogens. However, when carbohydrate was restricted to a very low level (about 15g a day), these elevated oestrogen hormone levels showed a definite reduction in both men and women; our measurements also showed that these hormone levels rose again if this dietary measure was abandoned. For detailed results, I refer readers to the article we published together (Lutz & Iselstöger 1960).

(Incidentally, we were measuring oestrogens from the adrenal cortex found in urinary excretion. Techniques of analysing sex hormone levels have become a lot more sophisticated since those days, and it would be valuable to repeat such readings nowadays. Given the good (but subjective) reports from my patients of improved sexual health over a great many years since then, it would also be informative to do this experiment with the slightly increased amount of carbohydrate that came to be my most usual recommendation.)

Sex hormone production is secondary for the adrenal cortex (the outer layer of the adrenal glands), the main concern of which is the production of the 'flight or fight' hormones: adrenalin and cortisol and, in this connection, I made an unexpected observation. This was about striae – the purplish stretch marks one sometimes sees on the abdomens of pregnant women. These marks are characteristic of Cushing's syndrome and are usually seen as a sign of hyperactivity of the adrenal glands. Now, many obese adults had striae, but I noticed that stretch marks were also often present on the chest, abdomen or buttocks of many of my obese adolescents. That the adrenals were indeed implicated, I was able to show by clinical demonstration that increased metabolites of endogenous cortisol were excreted in the urine of patients exhibiting striae.

So here we had another possible part of the jigsaw: just as I had found overly raised insulin secretion in the obese youngsters, now it seemed that overly raised adrenal activity was also linked to the level of carbohydrate consumed. Interestingly these striae seemed to appear only after puberty. Was there a connection with sex hormones, too, I wondered? In this regard, I had noted that very fat children not only seemed to have smaller genitals but also a delay in puberty: the more so, the greater the obesity.

Through clinical tests, I was able to demonstrate not raised levels, as I had found with obese adults, but a diminution in the normal levels of sex hormones* in many of these children. This was all very thought provoking.

Perhaps I ought to explain here a little more of the gland-based mechanism which regulates the sugar in our bloodstream, for there is a whole hormonal 'sugar squad' set up to keep our blood sugar in bounds, of which insulin and cortisol are the main players. The task of getting rid of excess sugar falls to insulin, as already told, aided by the growth hormone which, by suppressing the mobilisation of fat for energy use, allows the work of insulin to be prioritised. As the use of sugar is less energy-efficient than the use of fat, more cortisol and more of the thyroid hormones T^3 and T^4 are then called on to aid in the production of energy from sugar.

Should the sugar in the blood fall too low because, say of an excess of insulin, then there are three hormones to remedy this. Firstly, there is glucagon (the antagonist of insulin from the pancreas) to convert the limited store of glycogen (kept in the liver and muscles for emergency use) back into sugar; secondly, there is adrenalin (from the adrenal glands) which performs the same function; thirdly and importantly, there is the hormone cortisol (also from the adrenals) to break down protein to supply sugar to the blood, again should there be a pressing need because of a shortfall.

A doctor does not – and cannot – run his medical practise like a formal clinical trial. Though I managed to do a few research projects with colleagues, of necessity many of my observations are just that: observations based on evidence gathered during my ordinary day-to-day work with patients.

That being said, about this time I came up with a fascinating hypothesis, for I had noticed that, with puberty, obese adolescents who were still eating a high carbohydrate diet, tended to show a whole cluster of symptoms of metabolic disturbance. I felt the connections here were striking enough to suggest that what I saw as carbohydrate overload led to a definite syndrome, which I dubbed: 'the endocrine syndrome of adipose youth', and wrote an article of that title (Lutz 1964). This cluster comprised raised insulin levels and disturbed sex hormone levels, together with a depressed level of growth hormone and elevated levels of adrenal and thyroid hormones. I was gathering important evidence of what I came to see as the 'carbohydrate effect', by which I mean the serious detriment to our health of carbohydrate overload.

Conversely, I was also gathering further evidence of the therapeutic value of carbohydrate restriction. For example, once on a low enough carbohydrate diet, the striae of both adults and teenagers gradually faded*. Furthermore, two seemingly opposed conditions had also benefited: namely obese adults had shown a definite decrease in (already raised) sex hormone levels and, on the other hand, adipose youths had shown a probable increase in (already depressed) sex hormone levels. I say 'probable' because, despite their previous measurably low levels of sex hormones, once these adolescents were following the very low carbohydrate regimen described above, puberty soon came; it was striking how they then coped with this important change in a far easier and more natural way than did many of their peers still eating a high carbohydrate diet.

What interested me in particular was how, as these youngsters continued on the diet and their obesity lessened and they regained a more satisfactory shape, it was not just one hormonal level in the cluster that tended to improve, but it seemed to me that all the various symptoms of endocrine disturbance these teenagers exhibited gradually responded favourably. It was a milestone in this early stage of my journey.

A gradual changeover

My third lesson came about in the following manner. I was impatient to share my new experiences and, buoyed up by my results so far, I soon felt the need to convince my medical colleagues of the correctness of my basic idea – the curative value of carbohydrate restriction. This I felt I could only do if I could show its successful application to a disease that, so far, was thought incurable. Thinking carbohydrate restriction might be helpful in treating nervous system diseases, I opted for multiple sclerosis, for which there was so far no treatment that got to the root of the problem.

Nerve fibres are a bit like telephone wires, carrying messages to and from all parts of the body; some are of considerable length. Around these elongated nerve fibres is a wrapping made out of myelin, a type of fatty material which serves as insulation and to increase the speed of message transmission. In multiple sclerosis, there are pathological alterations in this myelin sheath, which I felt might benefit from a diet that brought about a positive change in the quality of body fats*; at the very least, it might slow down the destructive processes that were gradually happening.

I was soon to set up a study with a colleague, the late Professor Dr K Eckel, head of the Neurology Department at Bad Ischl, Upper Austria. It was the first medical condition that I subjected to systematic investigation. We took 36 multiple sclerosis patients, whose diagnoses, ranging from long-standing to very recent, appeared to be confirmed by clinical findings as well as by the course of the disease. Carbohydrate restriction apart, we put no pressure on the participants as to the ratio of fat to protein and we gave the patients a lot of choice as to what they ate. These patients were eager to be put straight on to the same ultra-low (15 – 20g) carbohydrate diet that I used initially with my obese patients. In fact, some were so eager that they plunged right into the dietary change before everything was properly set up. However, we soon got things organised. Monitoring was easier when patients were hospitalised but, through regular supervision, we were able to witness the willing cooperation of those at home and so confirm strict adherence to the diet.

The fact that multiple sclerosis is so subject to remission and relapse (and that even cases of total remission are not unknown) can make results difficult to assess. Nevertheless a clear pattern of response to the diet was discernable. With people who had been recently diagnosed (less than six months) the results were very positive: namely, we found that these patients were consistently helped by the diet. Those who had had the condition less than five years and whose illness came in stages, also often gained full or almost full remission; at the very least they improved to the stage they were at before the last downhill step. There were even a few 'miracle cures' – patients who 'took up their beds and walked' or rather put their sticks in a corner and walked. (Some of these kept to the diet and even years later were still free from relapse.)

There was, however, a conspicuous lack of success in patients with a long-standing condition of five years or more or who were already experiencing progressive and continual decline. It seemed that for those patients very ill already, such a low amount of carbohydrate was inappropriate; although some only experienced temporary difficulties, others had to abandon the diet altogether as, sadly, their condition worsened and some suffered an increased spasticity in their limbs.

What all this brought home to me was how difficult it was for someone seriously ill to make a sudden and radical change from one type of nutritional base to another very different one. Perhaps the nervous system was particularly susceptible in this respect and unable to adjust quickly enough to a major change in fuel supply? I did not know; nor in those days was I aware of the immune complications that tend to accompany multiple sclerosis.

Whatever the reason, my observations underlined the need for caution and for very slow change in dietary habits. It was a hard lesson but an important one, for it taught me the paramount importance of a GRADUAL CHANGEOVER FOR ANY SERIOUSLY ILL

PERSON, not just for multiple sclerosis, but WHATEVER THEIR AILMENT. After all my subsequent years of experience, I still hold to the need for a slow transition in such cases, a rule I also apply to all those in the 'at risk' age groups and to the elderly. Moreover, in certain cases, it is important not to reduce carbohydrates below a specific amount, as this, too, can bring about unnecessary complications and may cause people to abandon the diet before they have had a chance to reap the benefits – all points to which I will return.

We had made a start with our trial in February 1959. In America, in the autumn of the following year, Sawyer (1960) had reported success in treating multiple sclerosis with oral diabetic medication in conjunction with the diet for diabetes usual at the time. This was interesting as, by then, Professor Dr Eckel and I had been working for about the same amount of time with a diabetic-type diet yet without any medication. Therefore, though our study was small, we decided to write up and publish our own observations (Eckel & Lutz, 1961).

As the reader can see, things did not go as smoothly and simply as I had hoped: whilst some patients thrived on such a low amount of carbohydrate, it was certainly the case that not all patients benefited in terms of the course of the disease. Consequently, it was not long before I abandoned such a radical approach in favour of a more graduated one. Nor was it long before I, too, abandoned such severe carbohydrate restriction on myself. In 1962, my four-year cereal-free ultra-low carbohydrate trial came to an end: I upped my own carbohydrates and began living on the more moderate diet to which I have kept more or less ever since.

Reassurance

I have talked about the possibility of transitional problems, but another concern was becoming apparent. For it was during these very early years of using carbohydrate restriction in my medical practice – the late 1950s – that the idea was gaining ground that arteriosclerosis was caused by eating saturated fat, and especially by eating foods containing cholesterol. Both these substances are found in animal food, the very food that I was recommending.

This made some patients anxious and the worry that I saw in their faces ran something like this: 'I feel fine now on your diet, Dr Lutz, but . . .' I knew the 'but' meant: 'am I storing up trouble for myself in the long term? Will the diet raise the cholesterol level in my blood, the cholesterol then attaching itself to the arterial walls, with the much publicized alarming consequences?' I obviously wanted to allay any such fears or uneasiness. In any case, I would not knowingly put my patients at risk, nor would I willingly swap one disease for another – a point about which I felt very strongly.

As long as my patients stuck to the time-honoured natural fats, I was not personally worried by the fat content of the diet that I was advising. After all, if my evolutionary history were correct, prior to carbohydrates, fat had been our main energy source for so many millennia that it was extremely unlikely that animal fats were the cause of any real harm: in my view, it was far more likely that carbohydrates were doing the damage! Moreover, if the cholesterol-containing plaques that formed in the arteries were a repair mechanism, might not a diet that brought about such beneficial changes in tissue quality prevent such repair-needing degenerative changes happening to the arteries in the first place? This was how I reasoned.

Nevertheless, there was a niggling doubt at the back of my mind. Short-term benefits could be readily observed and were already often apparent, but I was proposing a way of eating for the long term. Was there a possibility of slow and insidious change happening over the years, unbeknown both to myself and to my patients, which might increase their risk of eventual heart attacks and strokes? But how to check this out?

(Here I must stress that the presence of arteriosclerosis does not mean one will necessarily have a heart attack or stroke, for these can occur when arteriosclerosis is only slight and yet, in people with severe arteriosclerosis, thrombotic complications may be completely absent. However, even if heart attacks and strokes do not always follow, arteriosclerosis is seen as a big so-called risk factor: namely a likely antecedent to such misfortunes.)

Now it would take far too many years to patiently await the absence of arteriosclerosis I hoped to see in patients on my diet. Nor could I wait for the consensus of medical opinion to come to my rescue. The only way forward was to instigate my own research.

I had learned from an article on atherosclerosis* in hens, written in 1956 by two German scientists: Professor Dr Günther Weitzel of Tübingen and Professor Dr Eckhard Buddecke of Münster that, though standing a long way from humans on the evolutionary chain, hens suffered from a similar type of arteriosclerosis to that which occurs in humans. Like us, they often exhibited marked arteriosclerosis in their old age (in the case of hens, their third or fourth year); prior to that, there would be a gradual integration of fats into the inner walls of some of the arteries, these deposits of cholesterol and other fats being similar to those in humans in location, in fine tissue type and reaction, and in chemical composition. Hens were also inexpensive, easily available and short-lived, which meant I could study the process speeded up, as it were.

There was a further similarity that interested me: that from having been more or less carnivorous in the wild, our domesticated fowl received increasing amounts of carbohydrate in their diet and nowadays lived to a large extent on grain – not too unlike the story of our own humankind, perhaps? Were hens suffering from one of the consequences of being led away from their original mode of nutrition, as I suspected we humans were? I approached Professor Weitzel with this idea and found a ready listener. I had to fund any experiments largely from my own pocket, so was grateful when he generously placed at my disposal both his own experience and the facilities of his Institute. I was also grateful to Professor Buddecke who lent me his assistance in the continuation and completion of the experiments, and for the financial assistance later provided by local firms, as well as from the governing body of the province of Salzburg.

This enabled me to set up chicken feeding trials to examine the role of carbohydrate (and incidentally of fat) in the genesis of arteriosclerosis, which, with preparation and writing up, were to take almost ten years. Groups of chickens – I picked Rhode Island Reds for the trials, choosing as pure a strain as I could to minimise genetic variation and selecting female birds that were equal in age – were to be fed different proportions of carbohydrate, protein and fat: the birds with the highest ration of carbohydrate receiving the lowest amount of fat and vice versa. The content of the feed was precisely calculated by Professor W. Wirths of the Max Plank Institute for Nutritional Physiology in Dortmund, food intake was strictly measured throughout the experiments and care was taken to ensure adequate vitamins and minerals. No limit was placed on calories, the birds taking as much feed they wished, and the birds were given room to roam.

All the feed given was natural, mostly from animal sources and the fat mostly saturated: all birds were fed a basic mixture of dried yeast, shrimps, white cheese and skimmed milk, which was mixed so that the birds could not pick and choose, say just shrimps. In addition, my experimental (low carbohydrate) birds also received meat but no grain, whereas the (high carbohydrate) controls received wheat grain but no meat. We were deliberately careful to limit both plant proteins and unsaturated fat, so that the outcome of the trials could not be wrongly ascribed to their influence.

The preliminary trial of two groups took place from

1961--4, the full trial with six groups from 1964--7. Differences between the two groups soon emerged: my (low carbohydrate) group grew more slowly, had finer plumage and appeared to have more muscle and less fat than the controls, and they stayed fit and slim as they grew older – that is if you can call hens 'slim'. In our trials, as indices of arteriosclerosis we concentrated on the amount of fat in the main artery walls and the formation of so-called plaques. In the first trial, an early examination by Professor Weitzel found that, after two years, in some of the birds the arteriosclerotic process had already begun and that, in spite of eating more animal fat – and remember it was mostly saturated fat – a lot less fat had found its way into the walls of the aortas of my (low carbohydrate) hens than into those of the control group.

The experimental set-up was far from perfect and there were some teething troubles. Nevertheless, when the hens were examined after the full three years of both trials, pronounced atheroma was found in some of the (high carbohydrate) control group. Frau G. Andresen of Tübingen, who was very experienced in such work, did the visual analyses. I remember her saying to me: "Dr Lutz, I have examined the aortas of many thousands of chickens and, in all the years I have being doing my job, I have never seen these blood vessels with less arteriosclerosis in them. In fact, I have never seen chickens with such healthy arteries as those of your own (low carbohydrate) hens!"

In order to compare the results of the visual examination, the severity of the arteriosclerosis was expressed on a scale of 0 to 6, with 0 showing no obvious degenerative change and 6, severe arteriosclerosis. If we add the figures from both trials together, they averaged: 0.8 for my own group and 3.3 for the controls, showing that there was far less arteriosclerosis in my (low carbohydrate) hens. The biochemical analyses confirmed the pronouncement of the visual inspection – that there was clearly more deposition of fats in the artery walls of the (high carbohydrate) control group than of the other groups, and clearly more arteriosclerosis.

The results of the trials were independently analysed and found to be statistically viable by staff at Tübingen University. Further details of the trials are given in an article in the *Zeitschrift für Ernährungswissenschaft* (journal of nutritional science) that I subsequently wrote with Professor Buddecke and Frau Andresen (Lutz, Andresen & Buddecke 1969).

In terms of my own theory, the overall results were very encouraging: namely, the finger of suspicion certainly seemed to point at carbohydrate. It was also reassuring that the intake of fat bore an inverse relationship to the incidence of arteriosclerosis. According to the tenets of the 'fat theory' – or lipid hypothesis, as it is often called – one would expect the presence of more fat in the diet of the hens to augment arteriosclerotic change, so it was particularly striking that the results showed no such relationship. On the contrary, the **HENS EATING MORE FAT HAD LESS ARTERIOSCLEROSIS** at the end of the three years and, conversely, those eating less fat had more arteriosclerosis.

Judging from the results of my own group and the control alone, one might therefore conclude: 'the more carbohydrate, the more arteriosclerosis', or even 'the less dietary fat, the more arteriosclerosis'. However, it was not quite that simple, at least in any absolute sense, for the incidence of arteriosclerosis paralleled not only the carbohydrate but also the calorie intake; moreover there were also groups of hens to which we gave a medium level of carbohydrate and fat in their feed.

Let me be more precise. My own (low carbohydrate) group's feed consisted of 27.3g protein, 12.2g fat and 12.6g carbohydrate; the control group's 25.0g protein, 2.6g fat, 93.3g carbohydrate. Proportionately, my hens received feed with a ratio of 53% protein to 23% fat to 24% carbohydrate; the percentages for the second and third medium groups were 35:14.5:50.5 and 35:17:48; for the high carbohydrate controls the ratio was 21:2:77. On the face of it, my group were receiving a high protein, high fat, low carbohydrate diet, whereas that of the controls might be described as low protein, low fat, high carbohydrate, with the others getting something in between.

There is a tendency to mix up the significance of 'proportion' as opposed to 'amount' when discussing dietary matters. I know I have done so myself on occasions. So here a word about the misleading nature of percentages, from which it would appear that the low carbohydrate birds were likely to eat more than double the amount of protein than the controls. Yet, when we look at the average amount the hens actually ate per bird per day, it turns out that the lowest and highest carbohydrate groups ate almost the same amount of protein, with 27.3g and 25.0g respectively! This sort of error as to likely protein (and fat) intake, which is caused by percentages, frequently creeps into people's perception of low carbohydrate diets, and is why I always prefer to prescribe amounts and not relative proportions of carbohydrate.

Nor must one assume that because of its higher fat content, gram for gram, the low carbohydrate birds were necessarily receiving more calories. Yes, their feed was much higher in calorific value (523 kcal per 100g, dry weight) than that of the controls (369 kcal), and one might have thought that, with a much richer feed, the low carbohydrate hens would merely eat less overall and that the other groups would take proportionately more feed to cover their energy needs. In this way, calorie consumption would have been more or less the same between the groups. Yet this was not so.

It was eating not the calorie-laden fat, but carbohydrate that made the difference: namely the more carbohydrate the hens consumed, the higher their voluntary intake of calories. It was calculated that the low carbohydrate hens, which received 18.7% of their calories from carbohydrate ate 272.8 calories per bird per day, the middle groups, who on average received 42.3% of their calories from carbohydrate took 317.9, whereas the group receiving

73.7% of their calories from carbohydrate averaged 519.6 calories. Even after allowing for the extra calories needed for the difference in egg-laying between the high and low groups (see below), it still held true that the more carbohydrate in their food, the more the hens chose to eat in total and the more calories they consumed.

In other words, whilst the calorific value of the feed given to the control group was lower than that given to the other groups, the control group freely chose to eat significantly more calories in total. This suggested that it was not the amount of calories per se that was responsible, but rather that, since the hens were allowed to choose their own quantity of food, one could infer that the eating of so much carbohydrate was self-perpetuating, with the calorie intake incidental. (We did not measure hormones, but this did remind me of the insulin-led greater appetite of my obese youngsters before they went on the diet! Also, of the frequent reports from patients as to how they needed to eat less overall once established on my diet.)

That it was the high level of carbohydrate intake that was primarily implicated in arteriosclerotic change, with increased appetite and increased calorie intake as secondary factors, was a view later corroborated by follow-up work done by colleagues, as I relate in chapter 6.

As to the groups with a medium level of carbohydrate and fat, they did fairly well and certainly better than I expected. In fact, in terms of specific fats present in the arteries, no experimental group showed the lowest absolute values on all counts, with the group receiving the addition of meat and some grain doing better than the group receiving meat and fructose. Here it must be said that all these groups showed lower blood fat values than the (high carbohydrate) control group which was receiving the so-called 'normal' grain-based chicken feed.

A word on averages! The trials had indeed confirmed that 'on average' the arteries of birds on low carbohydrate feed were distinctly healthier than those on high carbohydrate feed. Yet averages obscure differences: namely, on the scale for severity of arteriosclerosis given above, whilst averaging 0.8, individual results for my own birds ranged from 0 – 3.5, with most on the low side. In the control group, some birds showed very severe arteriosclerosis, yet whilst averaging 3.3 with most on the high side, the actual range was 0 – 6. It was interesting that, though most birds were adversely affected by feed with large amounts of carbohydrate and little fat, not all were.

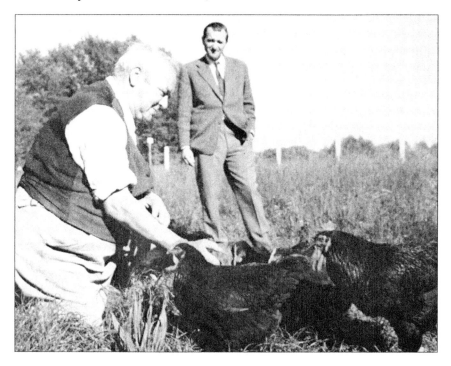

Figure 3.1: Dr Lutz visiting Mr. Fellner on his chicken farm

The results of the cross-over groups showed that there was more protective effect against the development of arteriosclerosis for hens receiving high carbohydrate feed for the first third of their lives and then switching to low carbohydrate feed for the second two-thirds, than for the birds which started low and then switched to spending the remaining two-thirds of their lives on a high carbohydrate feed.

From start to finish my chicken trials took almost a decade and, as we have see, there was a lot to learn from them. Above all, there was the reassuring result that a low carbohydrate, fat rich diet was unlikely to provoke or exacerbate arteriosclerosis – at least in hens! But the trials also demonstrated how averages can cover a wide individual variation, how percentages can be deceptive and words like 'high' and 'low' misleading, and that one should be cautious about jumping to conclusions by overlooking hidden parallels. Of course, I shall continue speaking of a 'low' carbohydrate diet but I refer to a diet in which NOT THE PROPORTION BUT THE ACTUAL AMOUNT OF CARBOHYDRATE IS LOW.

Lastly, I must mention a surprise observation made during our trials by my excellent keeper, Mr. Fellner, a real chicken enthusiast who, during his working life, had held a high office in the government and was now devoting his time to the keeping of poultry. I had told Mr. Fellner that, as one of the perks of the job, he could keep the eggs from my low carbohydrate hens. Seeing the lovely condition of these birds, I asked him in conversation one day how he had enjoyed the eggs. "What eggs?" he had asked with a wry smile. It turned out that, instead of laying eggs regularly (200 a year) like the controls, my own birds had laid 20-30 eggs a year, nesting just twice – more like they would have done long ago in the wild!

After years of carbohydrate-led distortion of the hormonal system of the hens, surely this was a testament to renewed reproductive health?

4   MY DIET

A modern 'Paleolithic' diet*

I would now like to introduce the diet I have used ever since those early days, both in my own life and in my practice as a doctor. It is the diet which, with certain modifications, I have used consistently over the last half century and with which I have treated numerous people with varying medical conditions. I have lost count of the number of patients who have benefited thereby.

When in practice as a doctor, I feel one should give as few 'don'ts' as possible; yet when the links in the chain of causation are understood and one can therefore expect good results from a particular course of action, one should be totally firm. Accordingly, I made the diet as liberal as possible in the things that mattered less, but was very strict about anything that I knew would make a fundamental difference to the patient's condition.

By this time – we are now in the mid-1960s and coming to the end of my stay in Upper Austria and my time as a rural physician – I was quite convinced that the carbohydrate content of the patient's diet did make a fundamental difference to the health of many of my patients. Thus, in keeping with my clinical observations so far as well as in keeping with my evolution-based theory, the emphasis of my diet was on the sufficient reduction in carbohydrate, together with the consumption of enough naturally occurring protein and fat, preferably of animal origin.

The essence of the diet was simplicity itself: namely that protein and fat formed its basis and, for the healthy, the only restriction was in the total amount of starches and sugars eaten in any one day. Otherwise, no item of food was forbidden and the choice of both menu and method of food preparation was left to the individual concerned, thus suiting it to a wide range of tastes. Naturally, during illness, there might be particular items of food that needed to be avoided, at least for a while and possibly in the long term.

I talk of 'my diet'. Naturally it is not my diet: its origin lies far back in the mists of prehistory! I like to think that its composition approximates to what all of us ate (in varying proportions of animal to vegetable matter) in those pre-cereal days. Indeed, this is the ordinary fare of many people today who, as a matter of course, eat and have always eaten the modest diet I recommend, as can be seen from the two sample menus at the end of this chapter.

I refer to 'my diet' for convenience and there is a sense in which, through persistent usage, I have made this diet my own. In fact, I actually wrote a book entitled *Die Lutz Diät* (the Lutz diet), which as yet has not been translated into English (Lutz 1986). The point is that 'my diet' is certainly less of a mouthful than to keep calling it a 'low carbohydrate nutritional regime with so many grams of carbohydrate daily and with protein and fat ad libitum'! From now on, the terms 'the diet' and 'my diet' will refer to the diet which I am now describing and which I regularly prescribe for long-term use.

I call it my 'Paleolithic' diet but, although I was initially inspired by the hunters of that period and, subsequently, was much influence by Stefansson, I have never gone to the extreme of an all-animal food diet. As has already been seen, I plumped in the end for the hunter/gatherer tradition of the slightly more temperate zones. I still held to animal protein and fat as the basis of good nutrition, but allowed a certain amount of daily 'gathering'. It was, I know, a compromise between what in theory I considered optimum nutrition and the necessity of implementing dietary change with real patients in the real world. Perhaps, if I dare admit it, it was also a compromise with my own longing for haute cuisine! Joking apart, there were many reasons for making such a compromise, not least that there was a long and genuine tradition of combining hunting with some gathering, especially when we move a little further away from the Arctic Circle.

As I did not necessarily exclude grain or dairy products, maybe 'early Neolithic' would be a more apt description? I have found over the years that, in the main, a mixed diet of both animal and plant food works perfectly well. My diet might therefore include some fruit, some vegetables, a little sugar and even some cereal, if tolerated.

Using modern ingredients, the resultant diet was easy, pleasant and satisfying and could incorporate as much variety as the individual wished. My patients might, if they desired, have one or two small potatoes with their steak or, alternatively, a few sugared raspberries with their cream! However, I will return to discussing the menu forthwith.

My Plimsoll line

What therefore was the amount of carbohydrate I settled on as my usual recommendation for a health-promoting diet?

In my books and articles when I talk about my diet, I generally refer to just one specific amount: that of 72 grams of carbohydrate daily. This was my Plimsoll line, if you like. This, for most people, was the target to aim for and around which to plan their day's food intake. This figure of 72g could, of course, only be approximate for it was not possible to ensure precise intake: not only is it difficult to make such exact calculations in the kitchen but nature herself varies in her provisions and so the starch and/or sugar content of foods will necessarily fluctuate. This applies even to apples from the same tree!

Nevertheless, given these provisos, this level of carbohydrate became the daily ration that, all things being equal, I routinely advised and it was roughly this level, which constituted the modest amount of carbohydrate on which my own family and many of my patients felt so well.

But things are seldom equal, and the treatment of disease by diet is no exception, therefore in no circumstances did routine advice override the importance of assessing the needs of each patient individually. For just as the ship's Plimsoll line could be a set of load-lines for different waters or conditions, so too did the amounts of carbohydrate I advise vary according to individual circumstance, as I shall explain in chapter 5.

The question of whether a slightly higher but still modest level of carbohydrate might still be compatible with health – and even work to prevent such diseases developing in the first place – was one with which I had little practical concern in my everyday medical life. As a consultant in internal medicine and so next in line to a consultant physician, I was constantly called on to treat people for whom a middle way was no longer an option. It was my view that a great number of my patients had already travelled so far along the road of carbohydrate damage that only a substantial withdrawal of carbohydrate could hope to start redressing the balance.

My search had therefore been for a general level of carbohydrate for therapeutic purposes, both safe and suitable for general application in the treatment of disease and for aftercare.

A general therapeutic level of carbohydrate

By this time, the reader may well be wondering about the importance of seventy-two grams. Why did I settle on this amount of carbohydrate as my general therapeutic level as opposed, that is, to sixty-eight or forty-eight or any other number? There were several reasons.

Firstly, it was precisely this daily amount of carbohydrate, which had stabilised Type II diabetic patients at the clinic in Vienna before the war and which had facilitated successful treatment by diet alone. It was keeping to this amount of carbohydrate – and no more – as their regular intake in the long term, which had prevented the degenerative changes associated with this type of diabetes. Note that 72g was a MAXIMUM AMOUNT OF CARBOHYDRATE.

With my own Type-II diabetic patients, I too found a similar maximum level of tolerance, with similarly encouraging results. Instead of putting these patients on a high carbohydrate, low fat diet, as happens all too often these days, I reduced their intake of carbohydrate to 72g a day, added fat and where possible discontinued their medication. This proved to be beneficial for latent diabetics, as well as for those in the early stage of diabetes where there is usually too much insulin and in the later stage where there tends to be too little. If weight loss was insufficient on the diet alone, I might also restrict calories. I found that, on 72g of carbohydrate daily, the fasting blood sugar levels of patients improved considerably within six months. Significantly, I found that both trophic ulcers on the legs and diabetic retinopathies responded promptly to the diet, with retinal haemorrhages disappearing within a short period. In fact, the better diabetes was controlled by carbohydrate restriction, the less diabetic angiopathy* was shown in the late stages of the disease generally.

Similar carbohydrate restriction was also beneficial for patients with Type-I diabetes. This type of diabetes often affects young people and is thought to be the result of a virus infection that destroys the beta cells of the Islets of Langerhans in the pancreas. Irrespective of food, insulin is needed for the so-called intermediate metabolism, so these patients necessarily needed to be given some insulin because their own bodies were unable to produce enough of it. Insulin, as we know, is also the main hormonal regulator of our body's response to carbohydrate. Obviously, the less carbohydrate is eaten, the less the need for insulin and I found that keeping the intake of dietary carbohydrate low and steady – again round about my 72g daily – was a very helpful measure. It made it much easier to regulate the quantity of insulin needed as well as the frequency of injections and so to prevent large blood sugar swings and the 'hypos' (low blood sugar episodes) that accompany them.

It was also round about this 72g level of carbohydrate, which helped my adipose youths maintain the headway they had made. These youths were not diabetic but as already reported, they did have a tendency to secrete too much insulin. Once their obesity was conquered and their blood sugar was more stable (i.e. the results of their glucose tolerance tests showed normal curves), I started adding in a little more carbohydrate and I monitored what happened, repeating these tests over time. The results of these tests showed clearly how 70–80g of carbohydrate daily was the most these youngsters could tolerate: once their carbohydrate intake exceeded this amount, the youngsters again showed the typical flattened curve of the hyperinsulinic. (See Lutz 1967 for more details).

I concluded that the best guideline for the long-term maintenance of their health was keeping to 72g as the upper limit, that is a level which seemed to give their whole endocrine system a chance to calm down, gradually eliminating the various symptoms of their 'endocrine syndrome'. Curiously, my Plimsoll line of 72g was turning out to be both a maximum and also a minimum amount of carbohydrate at which to aim. In other words, this amount was not only the upper limit for some patients but, importantly, I was finding that for others this amount proved to be the lower limit advisable, as we shall see in chapter 5, where I list precautionary measures.

In terms of my own personal experience, I had found that when I raised my intake a little – to 72g, that is – after my four years of stringency, the betterment of my general health continued, as did the improvement in my hip joints. Some of my adult (formerly obese) patients also found that this level of carbohydrate worked admirably for the purposes of maintaining their newly rediscovered figures as well as their reclaimed joie de vivre.

To show that it is purely the strength of the diet that achieves such results – rather than my persuasive personality! – I include a letter that I received recently by e-mail, via my German publisher, after the publication of our American book. Neither I, nor my co-writer Chris Allan had ever met the correspondent, whose name unfortunately got lost to me somewhere along the line. GERD, by the way, stands for gastro-oesophageal reflux disease.

Dear Dr Lutz and Dr Allan,

About four months ago, my boss gave me a copy of your book Life without Bread. I began reading it and have gotten through the first three and a half chapters. What is most exciting is how your diet has changed my family's life. We began in mid-August, 2001, on your 72g of carbohydrate diet.

Five very remarkable things have happened. First in that time, my wife has lost 30lbs and has been exercising with aerobic kick-boxing and has developed a great deal of energy. Second, our nine-year-old daughter who the paediatrician had told us was beginning to show signs of being overweight, didn't lose any weight but didn't gain any either as she grew in height to come back into line with normal weight for her age and height. Third, I had ballooned up to 198lbs, severely overweight for a man only 5' 7" tall. Since August, I have lost 24lbs. Fourth, in March I had been diagnosed with GERD and a hiatial hernia and was put on medication. Not only have I stopped the medication, but I have not had a GERD episode since starting this diet. Fifth, and this is the most remarkable, I have experienced a resurgence of my sex drive!

Thank you for your research and your book. I haven't had to give up any of the things I love (beer, ice cream, cake etc.), only cut back on their quantity and their frequency. We are also not spending any more money on our grocery bill each month either. We're just putting the money we used to spend on pasta, rice, potatoes and boxed side dishes into meats and vegetables. We've even eaten stuffing, sweet potatoes and pumpkin pie (in smaller servings than ever before) at several thanksgiving dinners in the past month. We feel great!

E-mail sent via German publisher, 8 Jan. 2002

I thank this gentleman for his e-mail but – lest anyone is tempted to do likewise and to try the diet themselves after reading only three and a half chapters of this current book – I would urge them to first study thoroughly the whole of this chapter and the following chapter on implementation and, if ill, to talk things over with their doctor. Remember this is an account of what I did and what I found when using this way of eating, either myself and with my family or, as doctor of internal medicine, to treat patients. I offer this, not for self treatment as such, but in order that readers may be more able to make an informed choice when it comes to compiling their own shopping list and subsequent menu.

Perhaps the most fundamental reason for the 72g was our ancient diet, which to me represented the 'ideal diet' for Homo sapiens. Studies of Inuit, who were still living wholly on their traditional diet, showed that the maximum carbohydrate content of such a diet of meat and fish was 50–60g. I reasoned that the carbohydrate present in the 'Lutz diet' was not significantly more than might be present in an all-animal diet: thus it was compatible with my idea of the best level of carbohydrate for the smooth running of our inherited metabolism and so most likely to be the safest and surest dietary guideline for all of us, healthy and ailing alike.

As a general formula to help those in trouble as a result of carbohydrate excess, my prescription was therefore not arbitrary. Just how extensive a range of disorders would respond to this level of carbohydrate, I was only just beginning to find out.

The bread unit

Now to some practicalities! In the Vienna of my student days, there was a popular white bread roll known in German as a 'Semmel' and diabetic patients were allowed to eat three of these Semmel a day as their total carbohydrate intake. For some reason, half one of these rolls came to be dubbed one 'white bread unit', which was soon shortened to 'bread unit'. In this way, these rolls came to form the basis of a handy way of reckoning the carbohydrate content of a day's food: namely, counting by bread units.

Now, as half a Semmel (weighing 20g) contained 12g of available carbohydrate (i.e. carbohydrate that the body can assimilate and therefore make use of), one bread unit was considered equal to 12g of carbohydrate. Six half rolls added up to the 72g allowance of carbohydrate – hence the ration of three bread rolls, which in turn equalled six bread units a day!

I remember that if diabetics wanted to eat something different as their filler, they were allowed to choose other items of starchy or sugary food instead. This they could do as long the total amount of carbohydrate these foods contained was the equivalent amount to these three Semmel, hence the drawing up of 'tables of equivalence'. This was an easy concept to grasp and this method of calculating was formerly in common usage.

Reckoning by bread unit is less common nowadays, but I carried on doing so to make it easier for people to work out their daily ration of carbohydrate, which I generally recommended as an allowance of 'so many bread units'. I always found it practical and my patients seemed to find it very helpful in their calculations. Hence, the fact that I commonly referred to my low carbohydrate diet as containing 'six bread units'!

The table of equivalence

The table of equivalence that I used with my patients is reproduced in Figure 4.1: it shows at a glance how bread units (BU for short) are used in practice. Sugar, for example, is virtually pure carbohydrate and is so easily absorbed by the body that 12g of sugar equals 12g of available carbohydrate. One teaspoonful of sugar weighs about 6g, so you reckoned two teaspoonfuls of sugar per bread unit.

TABLE OF EQUIVALENCE

For 1 BU (Bread Unit), you may eat the following:
12g sugar or starch
14g honey
15g flour, rice, oats, corn flakes, pasta, crisp bread, biscuits
18g dried fruit (raisins, dates, apricots etc.)
20g white bread, chocolate
25g brown bread, chips
30g wholemeal bread, dried peas, lentils, beans
40g cocoa powder
60g potatoes, bananas, nuts
80g sweet fruit (eating apples, pears, grapes etc.)
90g fresh or frozen peas, tinned baked beans
100g apple and orange juice (unsweetened)
120g acid fruit (berries, citrus fruit, cooking apples), lemon juice
130g carrots, leeks, onions, beetroot
200g string beans, aubergine, cabbage, cauliflower
250g beer (1 pint), wine (two glasses)
330g milk (full cream, semi-skimmed or skimmed)

Please note that most amounts are given as dry and/or uncooked weights. All amounts are approximate.

Figure 4.1: Table of Equivalence

White flour is high in carbohydrate, but as it also contains a small amount of protein, one got slightly more flour (15g) to the bread unit; the same goes for flour products such as pasta and flour/sugar combinations such as biscuits. Likewise, it can be seen from the table that one egg-sized potato of 60g (raw weight) or an eating apple weighing 80g would equal one bread unit. Bread is made in different ways and varies both in composition and in carbohydrate content, so the modern equivalent to one bread unit might be one slice of bread weighing anything from 20–30 grams.

I taught my patients to envisage all their food in these

terms – to 'think bread units', as it were. I encouraged them not just to weigh food but also to develop a mental image of the bread unit on their plate – say, of the size of one bread unit of apple or what two bread units of cheese on toast looks like. With practice, they became able to assess mentally the carbohydrate content of each sort of food that they ate regularly and could, for example, recognise as one bread unit's worth half a medium-sized banana, one medium-sized apple or pear, one small orange, four squares of dark chocolate, one tablespoonful of honey or twelve thin chips (French fries).

CARBOHYDRATE TABLE

Principle: Restriction of sugars and starches.

Permitted: Fish, meat of all kinds, including tinned and smoked meat, cold cuts, liver; selected dairy produce, i.e. butter, full-fat cheese, eggs, fresh cream, some full-fat unsweetened natural yoghurt, ghee, etc.; all meat fats i.e. the fat on the meat, lard, dripping; all oils and plant fats (though these are definitely not any healthier than animal fats); reasonable amounts of salad (lettuce, cucumber and tomatoes), leaf and stem vegetables (cabbage, Brussels sprouts, cauliflower). Salt in moderation (unless to be totally avoided).

Restricted: All carbohydrate-containing foods (starches and sugars) are permitted, but the total quantity of carbohydrate must be limited to 72 grams a day. See the 'table of equivalence' as a guide.

N.B. The carbohydrate content of mixed foods (meat pies, pizzas, hotpots, fish fingers, sausages, fish in batter, etc.) must be included in the daily quota, as must that of dairy foods such as milk and low-fat yoghurts and cheeses.

Figure 4.2: Carbohydrate Table of Dr Lutz

Instead of using bread units, one can of course reckon in grams, but I think reckoning in bread units is simpler on a meal-to-meal, day-to-day basis. Certainly, it is far easier to remember the amount one has already eaten if it is only a question of a count of six, rather than of remembering any number up to seventy-two!

The menu

I would now like to look at what people actually ate when they were on my diet. To give simple overall guidance, I would issue my patients with a general list of do's and don'ts in the form of my Carbohydrate Table, which they could take home with them and which I reproduce above.

As carbohydrates are found predominantly in plants, it is mainly plants (cereals, vegetables and fruit) and food derived from plants that have to be rationed. Therefore, though neither pasta nor porridge were banned, there would be a limit to the quantity of porridge in the breakfast bowl or pasta on the dinner plate. However, patients could freely partake of butter and cream and other animal fats and enjoy as much meat and fish, eggs, poultry and hard and full-fat soft cheeses, as they liked.

As the basis of a healthy diet, I recommended meat and meat fat (beef, lamb, pork, venison etc.), fish and poultry, as these were all nutritious foods and well suited to our digestive systems. I felt it was not imperative to eat any particular type or cut of meat, nor necessary to eat a wide variety of different meats. I remember the story, which broke in 1963, about Shirali Mislimov*, the so-called 'Oldest Inhabitant of the Planet', who lived in a remote mountainous area of Azerbaijan, and who was purported to be then 158 years old. When he was later asked for the secret of his longevity, he apparently replied that he had always worked hard and, for food, had never touched anything but chicken soup, cheese and yoghurt!

Preferences vary, in any case, and there was plenty of room in the diet to accommodate this. Some people preferred fish, others were not happy unless they had steak for dinner every night; many preferred to get their animal protein and fat from a mixture of sources, including non-meat sources such as dairy products; still others liked to take only fish and dairy products. So I left it open as to whether people ate fish, dairy products, poultry, red meat or white meat – I had nothing against any of these or any combination of these.

The important thing was to make foods containing protein and fat the mainstay of the diet in order that the biological needs of the body were satisfied, needs both for building and renovating materials and for an adequate supply of fuel. Here I thought it advisable to trust more to the sort of foods that had been longest in the human diet and to choose foods that were as nearly as possible in their natural state and which therefore had been least processed by man. This meant naturally occurring fats such as cream, butter, lard, bacon fat and dripping were therefore to be chosen in preference to hydrogenated fats, highly processed vegetable oils and hard and soft margarines.

However, just because a food was 'natural', did not mean its sugar and starch content could be omitted from the count. To initiate healing and support recovery, it was necessary to limit the **TOTAL AMOUNT OF CARBOHYDRATE WHATEVER THE SOURCE**. And, of course, one had to use common sense! I hardly needed to point out that it was sensible to limit, or to avoid, vegetables such as cabbage, cucumber, turnips, radishes and so on, if these caused too much of a digestive upset: there are vegetables that seem to be inherently 'windy'!

Yet, if well tolerated, my patients might enjoy a green salad with their plate of cold meat, a grilled tomato or two with their bacon, coleslaw with their ham, peas with their lemon sole, broccoli with their goulash or even the occasional Jerusalem artichoke, sautéed in butter and olive oil. Note that, since root vegetables and fruits contain variable and sometimes quite large amounts of carbohydrate, the carbohydrate content of these items also had to be counted in the daily ration.

Fruits are especially deceptive. I remember a colleague who, working according to my principles, was treating a patient for overweight and adrenal hyperactivity. After several months with no improvement, he referred this patient to me. The diet plan seemed in order and apparently strictly observed. Eventually, it emerged the patient was eating two pounds of fruit daily, which, though far exceeding the amount of carbohydrate allowed for the whole day, had been excluded from the calculation because 'after all, fruit is so healthy'!

The largest amounts of carbohydrate encountered in the daily menu were likely to be found in sugar, honey, flour, bread, cake and biscuits, dried fruit, pasta and other cereal products, potatoes and bananas. (I give these in descending order of carbohydrate content, as you can see from the Table of Equivalence in Figure 4.1.) It is surprising just how much carbohydrate some of these foods contain, especially in foods that combine many of these ingredients, such as cake, chocolate bars and breakfast cereals. I made it clear that it was necessary to keep a particularly wary eye on these. Snacks tend to be carbohydrate-rich: I instance the biscuits customarily eaten at a tea or coffee break. As for sucking boiled sweets whilst driving, that was tantamount to consuming pure sugar!

Many times I had to urge caution in the use of fruit juice, nowadays so popular and too often seen as a healthy alternative to fizzy drinks. I would instruct my patients that, even when unsweetened, fruit juices needed to be taken in moderation, possibly diluted by half, and their carbohydrate content included in the daily tally. The sugar taken in tea, coffee and soft drinks obviously had to be reckoned. Unsweetened spirits contain no carbohydrate, so a short before dinner could be discounted but not so the carbohydrate in wine and beer, which could soon upset the total aimed for, if taken immoderately.

Nowadays, such calculations are made easier for people wishing to follow a low carbohydrate diet, as lists of the carbohydrate content of individual fresh foods are readily available at bookshops and, as already mentioned, that of ready-made foods is usually given on the packet in the food information – a handy ready-reckoner!

As to fat . . .

I have always felt that food should be enjoyed. Yet, you cannot enjoy food if you are worried about eating it. In my opinion, there is far too much guilt around in respect of foodstuffs and this is hardly surprising in the current climate of opinion. I know that before going on my diet, some people felt guilty about eating dairy fats and so drank skimmed milk, shunned butter and, when tempted to eat a little cream, would look over their shoulder as though the devil himself was watching! I told patients they could freely enjoy such delights. Mind you, it was cold comfort to swap one guilt feeling for another – it was no good being permitted to enjoy fresh cream in one's coffee and yet feel guilty about that extra biscuit or that second slice of cake!

So, when patients came to see me, I would do my best to get them to relax about what they were eating and not to worry about the occasional overindulgence, stressing that we are all human and therefore fallible – sometimes one was bound to have more or less of a particular food than planned. I would tell people not to be too hard on themselves: if they did eat more carbohydrate one day, they should eat less the next. (There would then not be too much disturbance of the healthier balance that was gradually being restored to their metabolism.)

I would also try and reassure patients about eating fat. Here, one problem was that, by the time they came to see me, some patients had been trying to cut out fat from their diet so diligently that they were already eating an absolute minimum. As I described the diet I wanted to put them on, I would see worry cloud their faces. I would then explain that some fat was necessary in the diet to provide energy but advised them not to rush things – that it is not necessary to force themselves to eat more fat, but rather, especially at the beginning, to concentrate on slowly reducing the carbohydrates.

I would explain that carbohydrates can to some extent replace fat in the diet, as the body can not only convert carbohydrate to sugar but also to fat and use this as energy. I would also explain that this process can only happen satisfactorily when not too much carbohydrate is eaten in the first place, because otherwise the body puts a block on the use of fat for energy as happens with obesity. What was important was to first cut down on the amount of carbohydrates they ate and then learn to add in small amounts of whichever fat they fancied (or that they felt least distaste for).

As patients got used to this aspect of the diet, they started to relax and were surprised at how soon they managed to put back some fat in their diet without discomfort, and that they even found themselves positively wanting to do so! As their digestion improved and they began to see other positive changes in themselves, I would encourage them to add in a little more fat from various sources. It was usually not long before enjoyment set in.

Gradually, my patients would learn to sauté their vegetables and to incorporate the meat fat and juices from their roast into their now tasty vegetable soup. Eventually, such patients did not think twice about spreading butter quite thickly on their thin slice of bread, enjoying the fat on their steak or lamb chop, putting mayonnaise on their shrimps or helping themselves with relish to a generous serving of double cream on their small portion of fruit salad. For many, it was indeed a real relief to restore natural and once-loved fats to their dining tables.

This reintroduction of natural fats to the kitchen and dining table needs to happen or patients will go hungry. There is no question of achieving what some assume to be the 'best of both worlds' by eating a minimal amount of carbohydrate and a minimal amount of fat. Man cannot live on protein alone, and trying to satisfy hunger on a low carbohydrate diet with more plant and animal protein can lead to gastrointestinal problems, such as gastritis and diarrhoea. I have often been known to say that gastritis, for example, cannot heal in the absence of fat. In fact, if gastrointestinal patients on my diet do not make the progress I expect in spite of keeping strictly to my diet, the first thing I check on is whether they are eating enough fat.

Therefore, when living on a low carbohydrate diet, systematically cutting down on fat in the long term is by no means advisable – in fact, it must be guarded against. Fat not only provides the main source of energy, but it is also needed to provide us with certain vitamins, as well as to cater for various structural needs of the body. It is therefore essential that patients include enough fat in their food. Beginning to enjoy doing so is half the battle won.

A word more as to whether patients were likely to eat 'more fat' on my diet when, as they supposed, they ought to be eating 'less fat' than they had been doing. 'More' or 'less' are relative concepts: whether one eats more or less fat in total on my diet, obviously depends on how much one was eating before starting the diet. In reality, the amount of fat consumed by anyone on my diet will vary from meal to meal and from day to day, depending on the body's need for fuel, which would be increasingly supplied by fat.

In those earlier days, I found little research to draw on. There had been a great deal of metabolic investigation in relation to diet and obesity, but little on the likely fat content of a low carbohydrate diet. The study, which I did later with Professor Kasper and which I describe in chapter 6, was to highlight a wide range of fat intake both for the individual over different days and between different individuals (Kasper, Lutz & Wild 1979).

On my diet, there are several curbs to the quantity of fat eaten. For a start, fat is energy-efficient. Fat provides more than double the energy that carbohydrate does, so for the same energy output one needs to eat less fat than carbohydrate. Secondly, when carbohydrates are restricted, people tend to limit commercially produced foods and this tends to automatically cut down the intake of the so-called hidden fats (i.e. the sort of fats that have often been changed by man).

Cutting down ready-made foods leaves more room for the traditional fats that belong to our past: naturally occurring fats, such as are found in meat, milk, fish and olives. Once commercial foods are limited and these natural fats reinstated, fat consumption tends then to be self-limiting, as overeating it will make you feel sick. Just think of eating half a pound of butter with your boiled egg or small baked potato, or putting half a pint of olive oil on your small portion of green salad! One simply would not – and could not – do it!

Moreover, on a low carbohydrate diet, there is no insulin-led, false appetite to goad people into eating a lot of extra carbohydrate (plus the fat that comes with it). Once this false appetite becomes a thing of the past, the body will only ask for what it needs at the time and therefore little extraneous fat comes along unbidden. If we add the satiating factor of fat – for fat satiates as carbohydrates never can – we can see that fat consumption on my diet may well be quite modest.

Two sample menus

Here are two sample daily menus containing 6 bread units. As you can see, one menu is with bread and one without. The menu of any individual patient might be quite different: these menus are purely to illustrate the apportioning of carbohydrate, not to prescribe what anyone should eat.

Of course, the diet I have described in this chapter was not a blanket prescription, as this level of carbohydrate did not necessarily suit every person or every ailment. In the next chapter, I describe what I have found to be the safest ways of implementing this way of eating.

SIX BREAD UNITS A DAY

A.	Example containing bread	Quantity	Bread units
Breakfast:	1 medium slice toast	25g	1
	soft boiled eggs / cheese	Δ	–
	butter	Δ	–
Lunch:	lamb chops	Δ	–
	potatoes (uncooked weight)	120g	2
	green vegetables	Δ	–
Dinner:	roast chicken, cold	Δ	–
	mayonnaise	Δ	–
	tomato salad with olives	Δ	–
	French dressing	Δ	–
	2 medium slices bread	50g	2
	butter	Δ	–
	1 eating apple	80g	1
			Total 6

B.	Example without bread	Quantity	BU
Breakfast:	bacon and eggs	Δ	–
	half a grapefruit		1
Lunch	fish with butter	Δ	–
	grilled tomatoes	Δ	–
	chips (cooked weight)	50g	2
Dinner:	cold meat/ cheese	Δ	–
	garlic mushrooms	Δ	–
	lettuce & cucumber salad	Δ	–
	cold curried rice	1 tbsp	1
	fresh berries	120g	1
	whipped cream	Δ	–
	1 tsp sugar or honey	6-7g	0.5
	wine	1glass	0.5
			Total 6

Δ may be consumed in any quantity, as desired.
– contains a negligible amount of carbohydrate

Tea or coffee without sugar may accompany any meal.

Figure 4.3: Two low carbohydrate menus with six BU

Before I do so, I must point out that my diet could be as plain or – purse permitting, as fancy – as one cared to make it. Even on a limited budget and without overstepping the six bread units, there were ways of making things special. With a slightly bigger budget, there was no limit to the imagination that could be brought to bear on creating appetising meals.

In my book, *Die Lutz Diät,* I remember writing of a particularly delicious breakfast. It consisted of two cups of black unsweetened ground coffee, scrambled egg with crabmeat, one piece of crisp bread with butter and orange marmalade, and a glass of champagne (amounting to two bread units in all) – no wonder that, for fun, the 'Lutz diet' has been called a 'de luxe diet'! Guten Appetit!

5   PRUDENT IMPLEMENTATION

Making a start

I would now like to describe what I found to be the do's and don'ts of putting my diet into practice, the need for variations and modifications both in content and in carbohydrate levels, the various cautions I would urge, transitional problems that might occur when people first tried this way of eating, and its suitability for children and the elderly. Please note that, here as elsewhere in this book, I am concentrating on the dietary part of my treatments and will mention particular medical conditions only as regards the need to make relevant adaptations to the diet. Of course, I can only speak generally.

Let me begin with how I introduced the diet in my practice: that is, when a patient was sitting before me in my consulting room. I will have already taken a medical history and completed any necessary tests and medical investigations. I will therefore have made a diagnosis and have a fair idea of prognosis. This information enabled me to adjust my advice for each individual patient. I will also have talked through any measures other than diet that I thought necessary.

Once these essential preliminaries were over, we could begin looking at the diet. People needed to know what foods to give preference to as well as needing practical hints as to how to go about their calculations, so I always had by me diet instruction sheets to give out to patients, such as the tables reproduced in the previous chapter. It helped for patients to have a set of kitchen scales to work out the carbohydrate content of commonly used foods: diet scales that measure in grams were useful here as they measure small amounts accurately. I encouraged all patients to study these sheets.

If I knew a patient's customary intake of carbohydrate to be fairly large, I might advocate making a start by simply reducing the existing intake of sweet and starchy foods a little. This would entail keeping with the same foods but making slight changes in the proportions of foods on their plate. They might take, say, one less potato and more fish or cut a smaller piece of cake than usual but add a larger helping of cream. Occasionally, if I thought patients were well enough to do so, I might advise cutting carbohydrate intake to about half of what it was previously. For instance, I might suggest: taking one cup of rice instead of two for lunch and, at the same time, taking a larger serving of ham; still eating their beef burgher but with only half a roll; filling a glass of fruit juice only half full and perhaps adding water.

This meant that patients, eager to try this new therapy, could be actively engaged in making a start, whilst becoming gradually acquainted not only with the concept of the bread unit but also how it worked in practice: that is, they could begin to 'think bread unit', as explained in chapter 4. Since even a slight reduction in carbohydrate intake often made people begin to feel better in themselves, this tangible improvement provided an added incentive to continue with the diet.

Alternatively, I might advise people to make no changes in their eating habits but to keep strictly to their previous diet for the time being. First, they were to take stock of their habitual daily carbohydrate intake by weighing and measuring everything that they ate and drank during the day and night, everything, that is, which contained carbohydrate. This method had the advantage that people then knew where they started from and so could quantify the process of reduction right from the beginning – and feel justly proud both of their progress and of eventually achieving their aim!

Either way, once my patients were actively acquainted with their habitual intake of carbohydrate and with the bread unit as a way of reckoning, we would meet again to review the situation. Having taken into account various factors such as age, general state of health and what medical condition the patient suffered from, the next step was for me, as their doctor, to set the eventual target to aim at. After discussion, we would then plan together a strategy for reaching this goal. In this way, there was no indiscriminate (and therefore confusing) reduction of 'ever less carbohydrate', but a specified step-by-step reduction over a set period of time and with a periodic reviewing of progress to the target I had personally specified.

I found that it was often best for newcomers to the diet to apportion their bread units fairly equally over the day, allotting roughly one third of their permitted bread units of carbohydrate to breakfast, one third to the mid-day meal and one third to the evening meal. Snacks were usually no longer felt to be necessary once well established on the diet but, should snacks be needed between meals during the early months of the diet, these were to contain minimal carbohydrate and were to be based on protein and fat: for instance, snacks of cheese, cold meat or nuts.

Carbohydrate foods apart, I felt quantity, as such, should be left to the individual concerned. How much one feels like eating necessarily varies from meal to meal as well as over time. Our daily schedules vary, our ages, health and level of mental and physical activity vary and hence our requirements for energy. I would therefore give my patients the Carbohydrate Table set out in Figure 4.2 and, unless there were any indications to the contrary such as in certain cases of obesity, I generally imposed no actual limit on the amount of food per se that could be eaten. In fact, I assured them that they were free to eat as much as they liked of the permitted non-carbohydrate foods, together with any carbohydrate-containing food up to the daily limit of carbohydrate we had agreed on.

Once patients had their own customised plans in place and had made a start on the diet, I tried to ensure the principles of the diet were thoroughly understood by going through them again for a second time when they next came to see me. This was very important, as there will have been a lot of new concepts to take on board. It also gave people a chance to discuss any difficulties that had arisen so far, for most patients had certain aspects of the diet with which they needed help or points they needed to clarify. I was fully aware that it was not necessarily easy to make such changes. Indeed, for some this meant changing the habits of a lifetime.

After this, it was a question of giving the diet time to take effect and being personally available to patients, whether by phone, letter or in my consulting room, should they have any problems or queries. Here I must emphasise that regular one-to-one sessions were invaluable in helping patients through these early stages with minimal discomfort. Where there was SEVERE ILLNESS – and, in my role as a consultant in internal medicine, many of the complaints I treated naturally came into this category – I found that REGULAR PERSONAL SUPERVISORY SESSIONS WERE ESSENTIAL. Given its importance, this is a point I intentionally repeat and no doubt will do so again.

Temporary difficulties

The more relaxed and unhurried the transition, the more readily the body eased itself into the new diet. Done this way, for many the process of moving onto a low carbohydrate diet was straightforward and accomplished with relative ease.

However, after eating in one fashion for years and years – and one which was perhaps not the most suitable by which to promote health – the body will have done its best to adapt to what it received and in consequence will have made certain alterations in the way it worked to accommodate this adaptation. It was a matter of common sense that such arrangements could not be rearranged overnight. Even though some benefits might become apparent fairly soon, other aspects of the readjustment necessarily took longer and these were often internal adjustments not easily evident to the patient.

In the early stages of commencing the new diet, of course many health problems still persisted: namely, some conditions, especially chronic ones, took time to heal or even to start improving, other problems such as the bony alterations of an arthritic hip might always persist, as I was to find out myself when X-rayed in later life. (Here, please do not overlook all those many trouble-free years I experienced, even given the misshapenness of my pelvic bones.)

It is therefore not surprising that it was during the changeover period to the new way of eating that difficulties were most likely to arise. These were usually of a temporary nature. There might, for instance, be a lack of appetite for the new food combinations and this might take some perseverance as well as ingenuity in, say, creating suitable dishes that did appeal. Another teething trouble might be difficulty in limiting a particular food – fruit, fruit juice and bread were common ones – and sometimes it was easier to cut out a food altogether than merely to cut down the amount consumed. All too often, such foods were at first bravely reduced, but then somehow managed to re-establish themselves once more in their old quantity. I know it was often the amount of bread that tended to creep back up again unawares, slice by slice!

Even the amount of bread units tended to creep up. I confess that, as a family man trying to bring up children on my low carbohydrate diet, I myself overstepped the mark more than once, as indeed did they. We had to forgive ourselves any such lapse – this is all anyone can do! – and to try again the next day to achieve the moderation we were aiming for, possibly eating less carbohydrate the next day to make up for the overindulgence of the day before. However, the excellent level of health we experienced on the diet generally kept us 'on track'. Likewise, the unexpected improvements and new sense of bodily comfort experienced by many of my patients during these early stages helped them to know they were on the right track.

On starting the new diet, there could sometimes be physical difficulties such as a feeling of tiredness and the consequent need for early nights. Initial tiredness, even temporary exhaustion, was usually no cause for concern. The body was in the process of readapting to its ancient fuel combination, which, as a more balanced hormonal pattern was gradually restored, would facilitate more efficient functioning. Treated with understanding – which included taking adequate rest for recuperation whilst giving the new diet time to take effect – the tiredness soon passed.

Some patients were bothered with attacks of rheumatism for some time after the change over to a low carbohydrate diet, usually during or following a virus infection. In the main, I found it was enough to give a few prednisolone tablets (5 mg) for several days to bring this trouble to an end; occasionally, I have needed to give small doses of ACTH over a longer period of time and this, too, was very effective.

Now and then, there could be minor hormonal upsets: occasionally, for instance, the changes in hormonal pattern that came about as a result of the change of diet caused patients to experience a lowered sex drive, at least initially – I think I mentioned a case earlier. However, any loss of libido was mostly short-lived and tended to disappear within the space of a few months.

Another transitional difficulty that I witnessed from time to time was gum trouble, particularly in obese patients: the gums swelled, became spongy and occasionally bled. This, in my experience, was a passing difficulty and there was no need for alarm for the condition soon rectified itself as things stabilised. This was surely not a sign of vitamin C deficiency, as the condition did not respond to additional vitamin C orally. I think this extra growth of gum tissue was probably caused by the increase in growth hormone that tended to happen once less insulin was called upon and the various hormones rebalanced. Certainly, once well established on the diet, gums firmed up along with the overall improvement in dental health generally seen on my diet.

Probably the most common problem that arose when commencing this way of eating was that of changes in bowel movements. The movement of a healthy bowel is driven by peristalsis and does not need the impetus of fibre for efficient functioning. However, for those whose bowels had poor muscle tone to start with – the so-called 'lazy colon' – it was probably only the fibre in their previous diet that was wont to get things moving sufficiently. With the lessened fibre content of the new diet, this spur to evacuation was no longer present and the bowel might cease to move as readily as before. The result was constipation.

Constipation that commenced with the new diet was mostly transitory, usually righting itself after a time, especially when an increased amount of fat* was eaten. Meanwhile, if there was no contraindication, I found a little bran did not come amiss – one of the few occasions when I actually added fibre to someone's diet! Here a little experimenting could be needed to find what suited. One bowel patient, whose report I give in a later chapter, found that initially she not only had to strictly avoid all sugar, bread, noodles, coffee, black tea, raw fruit and fruit juices, sauerkraut and salad, but especially coarse bran and even linseed. A regular and soft stool was achieved by taking Kellogg's Bran Buds with hot milk for breakfast each day (naturally, the carbohydrate content of such a breakfast was counted in the daily quota).

Others found it helpful to start the day with a cup of espresso coffee. In my experience, it was women, more so than men, who tended to experience constipation when they first went on the diet, and particularly women who, before the transition, were already in the habit of taking laxatives. In this case, I tended to recommend that these should be continued, but as a short-term measure only, for it had to be borne in mind that too many laxatives, taken over too long a period, might damage the colon.

In stubborn cases, that is cases where the tendency to constipation lasted more than a few months, I felt the best course of action to be the daily enema, using one litre of plain warm water, for as long as needed. This I also advised for patients not accustomed to using laxatives and for those for whom bran was too irritant or coffee inappropriate. It was a simple and effective procedure but one with which some twenty-first century readers may not be acquainted, so I will describe it.

A so-called enema bucket could be obtained through a chemist's shop stocking nursing supplies. This was a small plastic container, which usually held between one and two litres of water and which was hung on the wall about one metre above the needed application. Connected to it was a plastic tube with a nozzle at the end, controlled by a tap. On days when there had been no normal bowel movement, the bucket was filled with warm water – about a litre usually sufficed. The temperature was to be about blood heat: comfortable to the back of hand and so not unpleasantly hot or cold to the bowel.

The patient then lay down on their side and inserted the greased nozzle into the anus and turned on the tap on the end of the tube. Gradually, the bowel filled with the warm water. The tap was then switched off and the water retained until the urge to defecate was felt. While waiting for the urge, some people found it helpful to move around a little or even do a few simple exercises.

The procedure was to be done in a gentle unforced way and should feel comfortable. For many people, once practised, an enema was easy to perform unaided, though some patients could require nursing assistance. Eventually, in nearly all cases, bowel movements would occur naturally without the aid of the enema bucket. Though I recall one very old patient of mine, whom I had saved from ulcerative colitis, jokingly writing to me that I had 'done him no good', as he now had to take an enema daily which, he said, frustrated him more than the colitis! Here one must remember that it is the hormones which speed the velocity of the passage of stools which are at the base of most maladies of the bowel, and that my diet tends to reduce the over-activity of these hormones – hence, for some, the occurrence of constipation for a while.

Generally speaking, within a few months, things righted themselves. This was the time it usually took for the tone of the bowel to normalise though I have known it take up to a year and, in rare instances, even longer as just told. Success was, however, nearly always achieved in the end: namely, the tissues that line the bowel improved in quality and the muscles of the bowel wall regained their tone sufficiently to achieve normal evacuation.

Slowly does it

When inaugurating a regime of carbohydrate restriction, I emphasise the need for regular personal supervisory sessions because the transitional difficulties could be of a serious nature. With any patient suffering from a serious illness or chronic condition, adequate monitoring was particularly necessary, as was beginning the diet very cautiously. Also, medical intervention could be required in the form of drugs during the period of changeover.

Experience had taught me that many of these difficulties could be avoided or at least lessened by taking the transition slowly enough and by making the reduction appropriate: I.E. BY MAKING SURE THAT THE REDUCTION IN CARBOHYDRATE WAS NEITHER TOO FAR NOR TOO FAST for that particular person and that particular illness. Just how far and how slow this reduction needed to be in certain illnesses, I had already begun to find out, as told earlier.

Hence my conclusion that the older or more ill people were, the longer they should take in getting used to the diet.

In fact, the reduction of bread units of such patients I felt should not only be VERY SLOW BUT ALSO IN STAGES, with each stage lasting weeks, months or even years. My strategy was therefore as follows: after determining how much carbohydrate a patient usually ate in a day, I would reduce their carbohydrate intake very gradually to a specified amount of bread units – and to no less than this – taking as long as necessary to reach this goal. Only after pausing at this level long enough to make sure the patient was obviously benefiting from the dietary change, would I proceed.

If all was well and there were no obvious contraindications to doing so, whilst still observing the patient's progress carefully, I would continue to reduce his or her carbohydrate intake, again in stages and by a specified amount, until the final goal was reached.

Please note that in any situation of doubt, I found it best to initially make ONLY A SLIGHT REDUCTION FROM THE NORMAL INTAKE, and suggest this level be maintained for a few months. Should an unfavourable reaction occur, no further reduction of carbohydrate would be made until this had disappeared; only then would I proceed with my practice just described of lowering carbohydrates by gradual stages and holding that level whilst attentively monitoring the well-being of the patient.

Higher than six

Together with the speed of reducing carbohydrate intake, the amount of the reduction must also be considered. In so far as I can generalise, I might, for example, reduce carbohydrate initially to say, 9 bread units – and to no less than 9 – and then, when I was satisfied with the patient's progress, by one bread unit a month to say, 6 BU. Then again, I might start by reducing carbohydrates to a level much higher than this. It would of course depend, as I said, on the situation. Judging both the appropriate speed and amount of reduction took skill and discernment.

In certain medical conditions, say for example after surgical removal of the gall bladder, I might eventually reduce carbohydrates to 6 BU, but thought it important not to reduce carbohydrates any lower than six. In fact, there were times when for some patients the reduction of carbohydrate needed to be halted at a higher level than six BU, sometimes temporarily, sometimes in the long term. In fact, it could be necessary to keep carbohydrate intake permanently at seven, eight or even nine bread units.

One reason for this was that a diet low in carbohydrate tended to strengthen the immune system. Overall this was beneficial and to be welcomed, but in certain diseases this very strengthening could cause problems by bringing about an aggravation of symptoms* before improvement set in; occasionally there could be prolonged difficulties and, of course, there were times when due to a worsening of the patient's condition (such as already reported in the later stages of multiple sclerosis), the diet might have to be abandoned and other medical treatments resorted to.

For certain conditions, this strengthening of the immune system was what I have referred to in the past as a 'double-edged sword', and this was where the timely administration of appropriate medication came in. Together with personal supervision and a cautious reduction policy, my own finding was that giving medication to subdue the immune system during the first few months of the changeover in diet helped make the transition smoother, thus guarding as far as possible against immune overreaction.

Here I am talking about those diseases characterised as 'auto-immune', diseases in which the body has somehow become aggressive against its own tissues. Multiple sclerosis is one of these, as is cardiac insufficiency, also conditions such as Crohn's disease, ulcerative colitis, rheumatoid arthritis and some types of asthma such as true bronchial asthma. In these so-called auto-immune diseases, I came in time to deem it advisable to prescribe MEDICATION AS A PRECAUTIONARY MEASURE. In most such cases, I would give cortisone temporarily in small amounts; with rheumatoid arthritis and heart failure, I might give gold* for a short while.

This graduated reduction of carbohydrate, together with careful monitoring and giving small doses of cortisone during the transition period, was the more moderate procedure that suited my multiple sclerosis patients so well. (Here I am talking about patients with a recent or fairly recent history of multiple sclerosis, for I had ceased to treat by diet patients in progressive decline or who had a long history of the condition). Once I adopted this method, results were consistent and setbacks or complications few: at the very least patients showed no further deterioration, often experiencing considerable improvement. To me, this confirmed the real value of treating early cases of multiple sclerosis by carbohydrate restriction.

Here I must emphasize that any big change can be stressful and radically cutting down carbohydrate can be just such a stress, especially in older people whose bodies (and minds) have been accustomed to eating a lot of carbohydrate. The point is that stress in itself can elicit changes in the circulatory system such as increased blood clotting so, for patients with existing heart and circulatory problems, I soon adopted the additional precautionary measure of prescribing aspirin for a few months during the transition period on top of my graduated 'slowly does it' approach.

Incidentally, this is the main point of contention I had with the low carbohydrate diet of the late Robert Atkins: that initially carbohydrates were cut too far and too fast, which I knew from my own experience of older diabetic patients in Vienna to be downright dangerous for some patients. In the 1970s, when his diet was under attack and he was called before a Senate

Committee, accused of causing heart infarcts, I went to see him in America to warn him of just this and to urge a more cautious approach. Sadly, my warnings fell on deaf ears. We did not meet again.

My own policy became to advocate a slow reduction in carbohydrate to anyone whose condition I felt might well be exacerbated by a sudden dietary change, and I would include here all those in the so-called general 'at risk' age groups (i.e. men over 35 years and women after the menopause, ages when risk of heart trouble is greater). The diet can still bring great improvement and even healing to people of these age groups, but I hope I have demonstrated that particular care must be taken during the transition period in order to prevent the occasional disastrous consequence. At the very least, the results of too much haste may not be the ones hoped for and might cause the diet to be abandoned before its many benefits became apparent. Skill and discernment are needed here, too. I felt then, and still feel today, that it is better to err on the safe side.

Non-patients

Prudence as to both speed and amount of carbohydrate reduction was, I felt, also called for with people who were not my patients. Over the years I was necessarily to receive a great many letters, which I always tried to answer as best I could. They were mostly from people whom I had not met personally but who had heard about my work, perhaps from people I had treated or who had read one of my books or articles and who were thinking of attempting the diet without medical supervision. Naturally, if their illness was serious, I advised them to come and see me, but if they intended to use the diet in order to combat what I felt to be a non-serious condition, I commended this slow and gentle reduction to a target initially higher than six bread units in order to minimise the possibility of side effects and give their bodies time to adjust to a different dietary balance.

Yes, I know that in my younger days I had been very impetuous and had drastically reduced my carbohydrate intake from one day to the next. I had been lucky: I had benefited tremendously and there had been no serious consequences. I am now an old man of 90 and in the intervening 45 years I have seen enough to know I had not been wise. In the light of my long experience in this field, I would say that, without adequate knowledge of the factors involved, 6 BU (72g) should be the lowest amount of carbohydrate to aim for, it being sensible for people dieting on their own to draw up a program of gradual carbohydrate reduction over many months, working slowly down to perhaps 7 – 8 bread units (80 – 100g), perhaps without any further elimination of carbohydrates for a long period of time, possibly for several years.

Even to the young and fit, regarding whom I did not have many qualms as to their attempting the level of six bread units straight away, I generally urged the same prudence if they were trying the diet from reading or hearsay. You see, we cannot know what damage has been done by the years already spent on an injurious diet, too high in carbohydrate – cannot know what insidious and imperceptible alterations have taken place unbeknown to us, so my 'slowly does it' policy is surely the safest way to change one's diet.

This cautious procedure – or indeed, even a lesser reduction in carbohydrate – could still bring many beneficial changes to health, as my correspondents frequently informed me.

Lower than six

When I said that it was sometimes important not to go below a certain amount of carbohydrate, I meant it was important not to go below this amount as a regular habit. Obviously, there would be days when people felt 'under the weather' and might want to eat very little or not at all, or they might not feel hungry for other reasons, such as an emotional upset. Then, it was only sensible to limit or abstain altogether from eating until appetite returned.

However, there were times when it was appropriate to deliberately reduce carbohydrates to lower than six bread units. For instance, some diabetic patients stabilised only at 4-5 BU and, to stay well, needed to remain on this level of carbohydrate fairly permanently. This was the case, too, with some of my hyperinsulinic youngsters, as I reported in chapter 4. For obese people who were not responding adequately to the restriction of 6 BU, going lower than six might also be appropriate.

In the main, though, I have not found much advantage to be gained by people going much lower than six bread units. I certainly could not put it forward as the aim for people who had already spent a greater part of their life overeating carbohydrate. In medicine, one has to start with a patient's present situation, assess the damage already wrought and, if possible, find a helpful way forward. Although, for some, a lesser amount of carbohydrate could prove pre-eminently suitable, I found in practice that I personally advised it to very few people. Clinically speaking, I only recommended going lower than six (either in the short or long term) if there was a special object to be gained.

Modifications in content

The alimentary canal is the first port of call for foods taken into the body, so it was hardly surprising that the digestive tract was often the first affected – or, at least, that parts of it were the first to rebel and draw attention to themselves when certain foods disagreed, though it must be said that this was also an area very responsive to the right change in diet. Perhaps one in three of my patients came to me suffering with gastrointestinal complaints. I found that relatively minor ailments of the stomach or bowels tended to respond fairly rapidly, but even serious ones usually responded sooner or later, for these were areas where an overload of carbohydrates seemed to bring particular disharmony into a set-up intended by nature to work smoothly.

Particular health problems, and especially gut problems of one sort or another, often required modifications in the content of the diet with certain foods needing to be avoided whilst healing was taking place. Patients would often discover for themselves which individual items or types of food they were sensitive to. Here I can only give an idea of the foods that, in my experience, frequently caused difficulties and which foods were to be preferred.

With new patients, once the necessity for limiting carbohydrates had been fully understood, I would then talk of the importance, not of avoiding, but of making a point of including some fat in the diet. This was important not just from the point of view of their energy supply, but because of the soothing effect that eating certain fats had on the lining of the gut. Certainly, margarine and foods fried in vegetable oils tended to act as an irritant: Crohn's patients, for instance, seldom tolerated vegetable margarines. My initial advice to anyone with a gut problem was to prefer animal to vegetable fats. In my experience, butter, cream, lard, suet and dripping were usually all well tolerated, as was the fat on meat.

Protein foods, such as meat and fish, seldom caused a problem. As to starchy foods, I advised patients with gut problems to take their ration of carbohydrate mainly from potatoes, or to perhaps eat a little white rice, as this was a cereal usually better tolerated than wheat, rye, or oats. Like with starches, moderation as to sugary foods was in any case necessary when carbohydrates were restricted. Some patients could manage a small amount of sugar or of fruit, but this was a case of trial and, unfortunately, of error.

Until they felt well again, I also advised people with troubled insides to avoid drinking coffee, which tends to speed the passage of food through the alimentary canal; in this respect, tea was found less aggressive. Wine, especially red wine, was also on my list of what to avoid, at least until recovery was well underway. If alcohol was taken at all, in my view, taking beer was preferable to wine.

Bread and fibre

Bread was a food that could be eaten in small quantities by some of my other patients without discomfort. To those with abdominal complaints, however, bread often presented great difficulty: namely, bread, especially wholemeal bread, tended to exacerbate their problems. I therefore used to encourage patients to abstain from wholegrain products, whether bread or breakfast cereals, if they were suffering from any sort of intestinal irritation or inflammation.

Thus, for some of my gastrointestinal patients, it could become quite literally a 'life without bread'. When their condition was much improved, it was a question of cautious experimenting and careful observation. But, even after getting well again, it was bread that was frequently badly tolerated and, if so, I suggested that bread was best left out of the daily diet entirely. As I have found myself, one can live very well without it!

One can also live very well without the fibre bread contains. Just as the need for bread is one of the myths of our time so, too, in my experience is the need for lots of fibre* such as bran. Yes, constipation needs to be overcome and bran can be a useful stimulant to a sluggish bowel but, as I said before, a healthy bowel works well without such provocation and much suffering can by caused by the addition of bran, both to an already overactive bowel and to its owner.

Admittedly, later on – long after recovery – some patients do manage a little bread. For example, a former Crohn's patient wrote recently:

> I still keep to the diet, but no longer quite so strictly. Sugar
> I can't manage at all, but I can have a very thin slice of

bread from time to time. I am able to eat 2–3 small potatoes a day and that goes down all right.

Q I, Darmstadt

This caution as to fibre also applies in regard to eating fibrous fruit and vegetables. During any condition that involves irritation of, or damage to, the walls of the intestinal tract, my finding was that FIBRE FROM ALL SOURCES – including fruit and vegetables – had to be used with discretion and its effects monitored. The same held true during convalescence. To learn of the distressing effect of reintroducing roughage too soon, just ask the experience of a patient who, on my diet, has recently recovered from a long-standing and debilitating disease of the bowels!

Infants and children

So far, I have mentioned mainly adults and young people, but what about the diet's applicability to infants and children? It goes without saying that nature intended babies to receive breast milk. Once weaned, however, I have always contended that young children should be considered as adults with regard to diet. After all, apart from mother's milk, primitive man could offer his children only the same type of food as he ate himself!

In my own medical practice, I included small children in my nutritional program right from the start; this, I felt, was the best way of ensuring that they had all the building blocks and other substances necessary to their growing bodies. In fact, there was good reason for the mother herself to be on my diet and the sooner begun the better. It could still be beneficial to commence carbohydrate restriction during pregnancy, but the best precaution to ensure the health of a child is surely for both parents (or better still previous generations) to have adopted a low carbohydrate diet well before the child was conceived.

Mother's milk, as I said, is the natural food for babies. I understood human milk to contain mostly water, together with 1 to 2 % protein, 7 % carbohydrate and 4 % fat, though in nature proportions do, of course, vary a little. Should no mother's milk be available to an infant, for whatever reason, and an alternative feed had to be made up, then I felt it important that a formula resembled the proportions of protein, fat, and carbohydrate in human milk as closely as possible.

Protein was, of course, essential but it was just as important that the feed had enough fat in it. Babies needed fat: without fat, they would neither be satisfied nor thrive. That being said, care had also to be taken over the carbohydrate content of the feed. As to adding sugar, it was important that formula milk was no sweeter than human milk; as to adding starch, in my view, starch in any form, whether given in the form of rice water, flour, semolina and so on, was a completely unnatural food for infants and only produced gas and abdominal cramps, as could fruit and vegetables, even in the form of juice. Then the baby screamed, the family could not sleep at night and the daily routine of both family and infant was disrupted.

Raising the carbohydrate content of formula milk higher than the 7% of human milk was, I felt, something to be avoided at all costs, as was the giving of sweet drinks. The last thing wanted was to start the baby on the chain of events that eventually culminated in carbohydrate-induced disease by giving it an excessive quantity of carbohydrate right at the beginning of its life.

Once weaned, young children received what I routinely advised for their parents: in other words, they received a limited amount of carbohydrate but could eat protein and fat according to appetite. Approached in this way, the transition from baby milk to 'adult' food was only one of degree. If one considered the matter, it was clear that the infant that had been wholly breast-fed was accustomed to food purely of animal origin. As it was gradually weaned, other foods of animal origin such as meat, eggs, fish and dairy foods were the closest in composition to the milk it had been used to so far. These therefore formed a natural progression and were usually well tolerated.

Looking at the transition from the point of view of energy source, a suckling infant derived some 30–40% of its energy from carbohydrate. As the infant was weaned onto solid foods of the type I have described, this declined to 20–30% and, once fully weaned onto a low carbohydrate diet, to 15–20% of energy from carbohydrate, with the percentage from fat correspondingly higher – proportions ideal both for its maturation and, in my view, for the rest of its life.

My own children

My own children were raised without commercial baby foods. Except for when they had some form of infection, when taking breast milk my children seldom suffered from stomachache. But I remember what happened when one of my babies needed treatment for a hernia and, at the age of ten weeks, had to go to hospital. Here it was fed a patent baby food containing 10% carbohydrate and, at the end of only a week, we brought the child home completely constipated and suffering from eczema. Once home, the child soon recovered.

Once my children could no longer be breast fed (about three months), they were fed on the following formula: 200g cow's milk, 200g water, 18g (= 4 level teaspoons) granulated sugar, 30 ml (= 3 tablespoons) cream containing about 30 % fat. This feed was boiled to be on the safe side, and was sufficient for two meals. This mixture saw them through the first year. During this time, my infants required nothing other than this formula, apart from an occasional drop of lemon juice to cover their vitamin C requirements (which I gave, since boiling the milk may have damaged its vitamin C content.)

At this period – I am speaking of rural Austria in the 1960s – cow's milk contained about 3.3 % protein, 4 % fat and 5 % carbohydrate. However, one cannot assume that milk nowadays has the same nourishing quality as milk from alpine pasture and mothers that cannot breast feed must rely these days on the advice of their baby clinic and health visitor when choosing a formula.

After the twelfth month, we increased the proportion of milk in the formula. At eighteen months, my children joined in with the family meals. Thereafter, the general principles of low-carbohydrate nutrition were applied and I am pleased to report that those of my children who were born after my 'conversion' and whom I therefore brought up on my diet – or rather attempted to, as far as was I was able – grew up healthy and almost entirely free from the usual childhood infections.

What did they eat, the reader may be asking? Well, they received exactly what anyone else might have given his children at that time, except that I tried to keep the quantity of starchy and sugary food low. True, I was giving them less carbohydrate in a day than many of their school-friends ate for breakfast alone. Yet, as long as there was enough suitable food available, they seemed contented enough and they found, for example, that a breakfast of ham and eggs (with only one slice of toast!) set them up admirably for the day.

We kept carbohydrate at a modest level but, as I admitted before, I cannot claim it was always as low as six. Nor did this mean that my children never ate a piece of chocolate or that they were deprived of the occasional piece of birthday cake or ice-cream, though sometimes I was probably stricter than my children liked! But, in general, my policy meant preference was given to foods containing less rather than more carbohydrate, so that they grew up without either a 'sweet tooth' or an excessive appetite.

How difficult it was, though, to get this message across! Here, I quote one of my patients who had for many years successfully avoided an operation on her bowel by keeping to a breadless diet of 5–6 bread units. In a letter to me, after saying how well she had been on my diet, she commented:

Unfortunately, I can convince hardly anyone about this way of eating. After years of doubts, which caused me much grief, my husband is finally convinced and his conversion has certainly lessened the friction in our household. My daughter-in-law is a biologist and her brother a doctor, yet she stuffs her two-year-old full of sweet things, fruit juice and carbohydrates and then complains all the time that the child is underweight, gets one infection after another and often suffers from diarrhoea. But she is not to be dissuaded from this way of feeding the child. I feel sorry for the little one, as I brought my son up according to your guidelines and he was a strong and healthy child.

E D, Vienna

In old age

I have, I know, mainly talked of my diet as an efficacious tool in the treatment of many illnesses. Being a doctor of medicine, the treatment of illness has necessarily been the predominant focus of my work and experience. Perhaps I have not made it clear enough that my dietary prescription – based as it is on our basic physiology, physiology that has been in place maybe 100,000 years or so – is eminently suitable for the healthy as a suitable and quite normal way of eating. For, in principle, any dietary pattern that is genuinely suitable for keeping our bodily constitution in good order has to be one and the same for all the family: toddlers, children, teenagers, parents and grandparents alike.

If someone has grown up accustomed to my diet, this is indeed so. But there is a considerable difference between being on a certain type of dietary regimen from babyhood onwards and beginning such a diet later on in life – just like there are always more potential difficulties in transplanting a mature tree than a sapling! That being said, with the proviso that one could not expect a complete reversal of conditions that it had taken a lifetime to create, my diet has proven itself many times over to be a very suitable diet for the elderly. By eating carbohydrate foods in great moderation, many of my older patients were pleased to experience a lessening of all sorts of different health problems – in itself worth achieving – and go on to experience a calmer, more fulfilling old age.

One of my patients started suffering from ulcerative colitis in 1964 and had passed through many doctors and had had many stays in hospital. When first admitted, he was poorly enough to need a blood transfusion and he remembers his first hospital meal: semolina with lots of sugar and cinnamon! Sadly, after discharge, his condition gradually grew worse with diarrhoea 5–8 times daily, mixed with blood or just blood; again hospitalised, he was told that only surgical removal of his bowel would help. He was unable to accept the thought of an artificial opening. The house doctor then pointed out to his wife an article in a medical journal issued by my publishers Selecta Verlag, which told of a doctor from Innkreis (the Austrian province in which I lived) who claimed in his book success in treatment by diet. In short, he then sought me out. In a letter he wrote to me some 30 years later, he tells his story:

> In 1967, being too weak to travel by car, I went by train to see Dr Lutz in his practice. After thorough investigations, such as rectoscopy, x-ray, blood tests and so on, Dr Lutz explained the diet that I should adhere to strictly. It was precisely bread, which the previously consulted doctors had described as very healthy, that was no more to be eaten. Total bread units were to be reduced to five. Fats, which had been described as harmful, were no problem and were allowed in sensible amounts.
>
> Likewise, all medication was changed, since no success can be had without this. We kept strictly to the diet – my wife, too – and studied the book thoroughly so that we could control the management of the diet better.
>
> After 2–3 weeks, my heartburn went away and the bleeding lessened. At intervals, I had relapses, at first in spring and autumn lasting up to two weeks, which then dwindled to a few days.

Since 1995, I have had no trace of illness and today, at 84 years old, I still feel well and healthy.

We still keep to the advice of Dr Lutz and we enjoy our roast pork without dumplings and we eat our cake, made without flour or sugar, with a large portion of cream.

D Y*

6   MIDDLE YEARS

Ten years on

The year was 1967, a full ten years since I had found the caves of Lascaux so thought-provoking and had consequently embarked on my fascinating journey of discovery in relation to carbohydrate and the diseases of civilisation. I was, I admit, amazed at my audacity in pursuing, even for ten years, a course of action, thought by both scientists and doctors to be utter nonsense.

Yet pursue it I did. The almost unnerving doubts of my early years as to whether I was doing the right thing by my patients were now behind me. I continued to apply my diet and the results of doing so provided me with adequate vindication: as one after another of our diseases of civilisation responded to the treatment, the number of satisfied patients provided me with enough encouragement to proceed.

I also continued to write about what I was doing, as I felt it important to go on sharing the results of my work as I went along. Articles appearing in 1957 and 1959 were the last on my scientific research from earlier days, after which I wrote solely on the new focus of my medical interest. By 1967, I had written several articles for medical journals on the observations that I had made in regard to the therapeutic action of my low-carbohydrate diet.

My first had been the article on the improvement in the urinary excretion of sex hormones that followed severe restriction of carbohydrates (Lutz & Iselstöger 1960), mentioned earlier: then came the article on using a very low carbohydrate diet with patients with multiple sclerosis (Eckel & Lutz 1961). The following year saw the piece I wrote about my own four-year dietetic experiment and also one entitled 'Arteriosclerose und Kohlenhydrate?' (Arteriosclerosis and Carbohydrates?), a connection I was already exploring (Lutz 1962). Then, in 1964, came my article on the endocrine syndrome of adipose youth. (This latter, you remember, described how, on a low enough carbohydrate diet, not only excess insulin but also excess cortisol showed a return to normal.)

By this time, I was treating with some success a growing number of people for gastrointestinal diseases. These included a range of problems from chronic dyspepsia and flatulence to more serious conditions such as morbus Crohn. That it was carbohydrates that seemed to disturb the production of stomach acid, for instance, (and which somehow encouraged its production even when not necessary, as in a fasting state) was demonstrated by the fact that complaints such as an acid stomach, heartburn or the acid reflux coming with a hiatus hernia, if not a symptom of some serious underlying problem, often disappeared after only a few days of their restriction. Due to its ability to reduce hyperacidity, my diet used to be a treatment for stomach ulcers; since the discovery of Helicobacter Pylori, a bacterium that thrives in an extremely acid environment, this is no longer necessary but the diet still serves as a useful back-up treatment. Perhaps it could also serve as an ulcer preventative?

In my experience, the response to carbohydrate limitation of what is now called the irritable bowel syndrome also tended to be fairly rapid. However, much time and patience could be needed for the intestines to reach a stable condition, especially for an ulcerated colon. In 1965, I had written an article on the beneficial effect of carbohydrate restriction in the treatment of ulcerative colitis, and now in 1967, I wrote a second article reporting on 40 actual cases of ulcerative colitis that I had treated by my diet.

The year 1967 turned out, in fact, to be a seminal year: it was the year which saw the completion of my chicken trials; it was the last year I was to spend in practice in Upper Austria before moving to the very different work environment of Salzburg; it was also the year of my first book.

My first book

By this time, I had witnessed the fundamental difference made to the course of a broad spectrum of diseases merely by restricting the carbohydrate content of a patient's diet. It was such a simple and effective tool for healing that I felt it deserved to be more widely known. At first, I thought to aim the book at the intelligent layperson, as the title: *Leben ohne Brot* suggests, which means 'life without bread'. The title was meant to be eye-catching, with 'bread' standing for carbohydrate generally and 'without' meaning only a little.

However, I was soon persuaded by my publishers to write it also with the scientific interests of doctors in mind, and therefore to include a lot of medical information in the book. As I wanted in any case to inform the medical profession as to which common diseases reacted favourably to low carbohydrate nutrition, I agreed. This was before I realised the extent to which the medical profession did not want to be informed!

Leben ohne Brot came out in 1967 and I shall refer to it by its German title to avoid confusion with *Life without Bread* (Allan & Lutz 2000). It was largely due to the interest taken in it by Dr Erdmuthe Idris that publication of my first book was possible at all. By Dr Idris considering suitable for publication the manuscript of a then unknown author, my work on nutrition and disease was brought to the notice of the German medical world. I am sure there will come a time when the anti-fat propaganda no longer prevails, and then the service rendered by Dr Idris and her husband in spreading the word about low carbohydrate nutrition will receive the recognition it deserves.

My debt of gratitude extends to Professor Weitzel, who wrote in the preface to the first edition of *Leben ohne Brot*:

> Previous attempts at reforming human diet came mostly from the standpoint that lacto-vegetarian fare was to be strived for. Now, Dr Lutz has made a striking entry into discussion of optimal human nutrition with a revolutionary idea. His starting point is that mankind lived predominantly on a diet of meat over the long span of time during which Homo sapiens was formed genetically. Above all, it was a question of the Ice Ages that lasted several hundred thousand years: in this time span, primitive man had lived almost entirely on animal food. Since increased quantities of carbohydrate have only recently become part of human food, Dr Lutz deduces from this that the hormonal secretion of the human organism is determined by a meat diet.
>
> Weitzel in Lutz (1967)

Professor Weitzel told how I had carried out chicken experiments in support of this hypothesis, which had shown that a mostly animal food diet brought about a protective effect in relation to arteriosclerosis. He wished my 'thoroughly stimulating book' wide circulation, saying that my ideas had given a new impulse to experimental research on nutrition. If only!

Anyone who has found himself in the position of an outsider trying to penetrate the sacred precinct of established scientific theory will appreciate the difficulties involved. As a research scientist I had been an insider. Now, not only did my ideas necessarily challenge the current orthodoxy but, as a clinician, I was working full-time with patients. In other words, I was not part of a medical research team in an establishment devoted to investigation and theorising, nor had I the funding available that such establishments could command.

I felt quite strongly that clinicians often had an important contribution to make both to research and to medical theory: they were 'on the ground', so to speak, and observations were made first-hand. Many useful insights were gained in this way.

Moreover, clinicians were observing the effects of their work – in my case, the effects of a diet on human physiology – not just for short trial periods, but day in day out, over months and sometimes over many years.

Perhaps I could illustrate the climate of the time by quoting what Professor Hans Glatzel, former head of the Max Planck Institute for Nutritional Physiology at Dortmund, wrote in his foreword to a later edition of the book:

> The first edition of this book appeared in 1967. It was a courageous feat, at a time when fat was held to be responsible for coronary infarction and many other diseases, to recommend the restriction of nutritional carbohydrate to 60 – 70g per day . . . Lutz stirred up a hornet's nest! In the ensuing years evidence from other sources and his own extensive experience have confirmed the value of his concept. 'Leben ohne Brot' has become almost a slogan . . .
>
> Even those who cannot entirely accept Lutz's concepts and hypotheses regarding pathogenesis cannot afford to ignore this book. Clinical observations cannot he talked out of existence nor should they be dismissed simply because they conflict with one's own theories. The value of a diet can only be judged on the basis of clinical experience and practical success, and does not depend upon biochemical and physiological explanations.
>
> Lutz's book challenges physicians to gather data on a 'Life without Bread'. It is an appeal to us to document results in the prophylaxis and therapy of adiposity, peptic ulcers, ulcerative colitis, hepatitis, arteriosclerosis and coronary infarction as well as to record our observations on healthy individuals who have taken up the form of diet on which mankind lived for at least two million years.
>
> Glatzel in Lutz (1975)

The 'clinical experience and practical success' of my diet, I agree, are still the most important evidence that I have to put forward in support of the way of eating that I propound. I also feel that, in this and my other books and articles, I personally have done what I can to document the 'prophylaxis and therapy of disease', mentioned by Professor Glatzel. Yet the challenge to other physicians to 'gather data on a Life without Bread', still remains largely unheeded even after so many years!

I live in the hope that the medical profession as a whole will one day take due heed of the value of carbohydrate restriction in both treating and preventing disease. Perhaps, given the phenomenal sales of books by Dr Atkins, this may at last happen, if only through the groundswell of public interest.

Three years later, in 1970, Dr Idris and her husband Dr Ildar Idris, and their publishing company Selecta Verlag, gave me further encouragement by bringing out *Internistischer Alltag* (the everyday life of a doctor of internal medicine), a more technical book addressed specifically to my medical colleagues.

I encounter Professor Jürgen Schole

By the time the full results of my chicken-feeding trials were published (Lutz, Andresen & Buddecke 1969) I had moved to Salzburg to work. Medically speaking, things are a little different when you move from a rural practice to the city: there was now more specialism and the range of conditions I treated changed. People with multiple sclerosis were now likely to be seen by a neurologist, for example, and obese youngsters to be seen by a paediatrician. Nevertheless, as a consultant in internal medicine, I was still pondering how my observations in regard to carbohydrate and the endocrine system could be explained. The success of my chicken trials in showing a link between carbohydrate intake and arteriosclerosis in hens had not gone unnoticed and my experiments were already attracting criticism.

An acquaintance of mine, a vet, told me that a certain professor felt that my method of chicken rearing did not provide rigorous enough scientific control, giving the chickens a free run, for example. Of course they found grubs and worms, but this was intended to keep them healthy. Personally, I disapproved of caging birds and thought it was better to keep hens in good roomy conditions. In fact, I was rather pleased that my experimental birds – those on a low carbohydrate diet, that is – had won medals at poultry shows for their splendid physique!

The critic of my chicken experiments turned out to be Professor Dr Jürgen K. Schole from the School of Veterinary Medicine at the University of Hanover, Germany. After an exchange of letters, Professor Schole suggested we meet in Munich. Though no biochemist myself, it was soon obvious we shared a fascination for hormonal behaviour, which proved the beginning of a lasting, if sometimes challenging, interchange of ideas between us, as well as the beginning of a life-long personal friendship.

Professor Schole and his colleagues had been doing detailed research work on the carbohydrate metabolism of warm-bloodied animals, focussing on the endocrinal mechanisms that regulated efficient energy exchange. Jürgen Schole himself was interested in the way the body adapted to stress and saw knowledge of the way hormones work at molecular level as the basis for understanding diseases associated with hormonal regulation, which, albeit from a different angle, was a topic of particular interest to me.

Now, here was a professor of biochemistry who was suggesting that THE HORMONAL BALANCE OF ANY WARM-BLOODIED ANIMAL WAS LIKELY TO BE UPSET BY EXCESSIVE CARBOHYDRATE INTAKE. You can imagine how this immediately caught my attention! Moreover, the hormones in which I had myself discerned a certain interlinking pattern turned out to be the very hormones that were central to the observations made by Schole. The depression of the growth hormone, the raised level of corticosteroids and thyroid hormones and even the raised level of sex hormones were, it seemed, an integral part of the response to a raised insulin level in warm-bloodied animals generally.

It is not my intention in this short account of my work to delve into either technical details or complicated theories about hormones. However, as our hormones are involved in one way or another in most of our diseases of civilisation, I would like to mention a few salient points, for Schole and I were not alone in our observations. In 1969, the same year as my chicken article came out, Stout and Valance-Owen wrote that they thought a raised level of insulin particularly responsible for the damaging changes in the blood vessel walls and, in 1971, John Yudkin echoed my own sentiments as to excessive carbohydrate being responsible for increased arteriosclerotic development.

In a symposium in 1972, Schole reported that keeping calories constant and replacing carbohydrate with fat reduced the tendency to a fatty liver as well as to arteriosclerosis, whilst increasing the resistance to stress, including infections. The reason he gave was that the reduced intake of carbohydrate brought about an adjustment in the endocrine system, lowering the insulin level and simultaneously raising the level of the growth hormone which latter, he said, was essential for the proper regulation of the immune system and hence the increased resistance to infection.

This interchange between insulin and the growth hormone is illustrated by the work of Lundbaek et al. (1972), who showed very clearly how this exchange takes place in children after being given 50g of glucose orally: at first the level of both hormones rose, but within minutes insulin continued to rise and the growth hormone fell, followed after about one and a half hours by the opposite, namely, a steep rise in growth hormone and a fall in insulin.

It followed that the right balance of fuel was needed to promote optimum performance of both these important hormones. This reciprocal relationship between insulin and the growth hormone is one of the reasons why energy from carbohydrate cannot be equated with the energy derived from fat: namely, that the effect on our bodies and on the behaviour of our hormones is very different. It is therefore very important to realise that CALORIES ARE NOT MERELY 'CALORIES' WHATEVER THEIR SOURCE!

Moreover, amongst other things, this balance between insulin and the growth hormone may prove important in the prevention and treatment of cancer. In his experiments on rats, Schole was to show that replacing carbohydrate (maize starch) by up to 30% fat significantly increased their resistance to carcinogens – butter yellow* in this case – resulting in a greatly reduced rate of tumour growth (Schole et al., 1978). The work of Haas (1984) showed that adding fat was not enough per se, and that, for instance, using sugar instead of maize made little difference: the rats were only less easily affected by the cancer-producing agent, if they ate some fat and also kept their total carbohydrate low enough.

I mention this because it is similar to my own observation on patients. It is my impression that in those patients who already had cancer when they came to me, once on my diet, the tumour growth rate was far slower than one would normally expect. Not only that, but I found there was less metastasis, for example in female patients after operation for breast cancer. (This topic is explored further in my books *Leben ohne Brot* and *Life without Bread*.)

Given his interest in the corrupting effect that excess carbohydrate has on the metabolism, Professor Schole wanted to check out for himself how this might contribute to the development of arteriosclerosis. He therefore decided to do his own chicken experiments – and to his own exacting standards! This he did together with Professors P Sallmann and G Harisch, using very different methods (for example confining the hens in a battery and using inert material such as talcum powder as a filler).

In their two-year study, Schole et al found that, compared to the controls given the standard high-carbohydrate laying diet, the reduction of carbohydrate lowered the prevalence of atherosclerosis in the hens and whatever the method. For this held true whether hens were given fat instead of carbohydrate (with calories held constant) or carbohydrate was merely reduced (this latter group had the lowest incidence). The results of these trials led Schole to suggest that arteriosclerotic changes were aggravated by calories from dietary fat only if these calories were taken in conjunction with a lot of carbohydrate. Note that:

> A correlation between serum lipids or cholesterol with arteriosclerotic changes could not be demonstrated . . . It is concluded that isocaloric replacement of carbohydrate by fat or protein lowers the insulin level and this reduces the tendency to arteriosclerotic change.
>
> Sallmann, Harisch & Schole (1976)

Thus these results largely confirmed my own observations as to the benefit of carbohydrate restriction in reducing the incidence of arteriosclerosis.

During our long friendship, Schole remained my fiercest critic. However, in the 1980s, we nevertheless collaborated on a book *Regulationskrankheiten* (diseases of hormonal regulation), which to date has not been translated. This joint book of ours was published by the Ferdinand Enke Verlag, Stuttgart; it was aimed at a scientific readership and contained the results of an extensive literature search on these topics (Schole & Lutz 1988).

In it, we focussed on hormonal balance and the effect that disturbances in the equilibrium between the catabolic and anabolic hormones had on our health – catabolic being the breaking down of substance to release energy and anabolic the use of energy to build substance. Schole, the biochemist, was looking at this from the point of view of our energy metabolism, I from the angle of human medicine. What Schole called his 'three component theory' about how the catabolic hormones, predominantly cortisol and the thyroid hormones: T^3 and T^4 balanced the so-called anabolic factor (at the level of the cell, the organ and the whole body)*, I found inspiring, especially in relation to the implications of any suboptimal balance for the creation of disease.

For hormonal equilibrium to be maintained, there has to be a reasonable state of harmony between the organism and its environment, since health always depends on the successful adaptation to stresses, whether these come from the internal or external environment, i.e. from inside or from outside of the body. (By stress, I mean here a stimulus strong enough to elicit an adaptive response from an organism.) Naturally, there will be considerable variation in the prevailing stresses that the body has to deal with. In the book, Schole and I suggested that the nature of stresses in our so-called civilised world were different from the stresses that humankind was subjected to in a state of nature in three important respects: firstly that there has been a comparative reduction in physical stress; secondly that there has been an increase in mental stress; thirdly that our modern diet is in itself a source of stress. All three factors we saw as having a significant and disruptive influence on the interplay between anabolic and catabolic activity in the body's metabolism.

Put more simply, too little physical activity, too much demand on the mind and emotions and the composition of the modern diet are all likely to upset the equilibrium in question. You can imagine how my interest was particularly aroused by the dietary factor, for it was the insulin response to an excess of carbohydrate in the diet that was alluded to as a major modern stress on the metabolism.

Against the larger backdrop of these three major stresses of civilised life and building on the work of Ludwig Heilmeyer (1953), the book sets Schole's ideas on the balance of catabolic and anabolic forces against the ideas of Hans Selye (1936, 1952) on the biological mechanism of adaptation to stress*. We used this framework for looking at how our metabolism can get out of kilter and for understanding some of the ways chronic disease can come about. Schole detailed the microprocesses involved in energy exchange and use, within and between individual cells and between the organs of the body. Thus most of the work was highly biochemical (not my forte); I wrote the part pertaining to imbalance at the level of the whole body.

Jürgen Schole was to give me credit for my own observations in this field when he wrote in the foreword to the ninth German edition of *Leben ohne Brot*:

> Lutz has identified and summarised very nicely the 'regulatory diseases', which respond to carbohydrate restriction. Furthermore, he was the first to describe the endocrine events that underlie these disorders. Generally, his view coincides with the basic metabolic regulation we have postulated based on experimental results.

I would like, in my turn, to pay tribute to my late friend, Jürgen Schole, as the one who gave cogency to these observations of mine by providing me with insight into the biological mechanism of hormonal equilibrium.

Whilst on the subject of my friend Jürgen Schole, this is what he had to say in support of my contention that excessive eating of sugars and starches was incompatible with the extreme physical inactivity of modern man:

> Glucose is essential for higher evolved organisms, as the efficient systems of gluconeogenesis and regulation document. These reactions maintain the blood sugar level essential for life. However, the surplus of carbohydrates combined with minimal activity can throw the finely tuned endocrine system off balance and lead to secondary false regulations. Whole tissue complexes can thereby lose their function; even minimal stress can lead to pathological processes.

This was in the Foreword from which I just quoted. I have already mentioned Schole's work on cancer-promoting agents. His findings and views are given succinctly in this same Foreword:

> . . . we were able to demonstrate that the rates of tumour growth in experimental animals, which follow the application of carcinogens, diminish significantly when carbohydrates are replaced by the isocaloric amount of fat. This can be interpreted as a generally increased stress tolerance of all body cells and by intensified immune mechanism, whereby

the developing tumour cells are eliminated more efficiently.

These results indicate that in addition to tobacco abstinence, low carbohydrate nutrition is the best prophylaxis against arteriosclerosis, coronary infarction and cancer, since adequate physical exercise becomes more and more difficult to realise in today's metropolitan life styles. The same goes for diseases of the gastric and intestinal mucosa, to name only a few examples.

Schole in Lutz (1986)

Continuing medical work

From the work of Schole et al, to those with ears to hear, warnings of the carbohydrate effect were coming in loud and clear, pointing as they did to the sometimes dire consequences of an overly raised insulin level, itself the consequence of carbohydrate overload. For my own part, I continued writing up in journals any observations of particular interest, as the quickest way of bringing the subject forward for discussion.

In the late 1960s, there was already a lot of talk about so-called risk factors, factors which signaled a greater likelihood of a person suffering a heart attack or stroke or other complications of arteriosclerosis. According to the 'fat theory', as it came to be called, a diet that was protein and fat rich was just the sort of diet to bring about an increase in these factors. I had to be concerned about this but, as long as carbohydrate was kept low, I was to find in practice something quite different than that expected by the adherents of this theory.

I have already mentioned obesity and diabetes. Another risk factor was thought to be an elevated level of the blood pigment haemoglobin (i.e. an increased number of blood cells per unit of volume); this effectively thickens the blood, which increases the tendency to clots. It first came to my notice whilst slimming overweight patients that this condition responds well to my diet: the haemoglobin concentration quickly drops and the number of red blood cells decrease. This reaction happened so regularly that I dubbed the common form of the condition, for which no specific cause is known, 'carbohydrate-dependent'. (Note: I do not speak here of malignant forms of this condition, which may worsen: please see my medical books or my article 'Kohlenhydratabhängig Polyglobulie' (carbohydrate-dependent erythrocytosis 1968). Serum cholesterol and triglyceride levels also showed a tendency to fall. It is of great practical importance that these and other 'risk factors' can be treated dietetically, as I spelt out in my later article on nutrition and risk factors 'Ernährung und Risikofaktoren' (1977).

By the nineteen seventies, from being a medical scientist, I had already spent over twenty years as a physician and over ten years using low carbohydrate nutrition therapeutically. I had already had time enough to witness the difference such nutrition made in the treatment of liver disorders. Now the liver is supposed to rejoice when fat is limited and carbohydrate plentifully supplied, but it is not so: namely, the liver rejoices over the Ice Age diet it evolved to expect and to work with. This was to be my experience with thousands of patients, whose laboratory test values I have monitored over time and the findings of which showed significant improvement in the great majority of chronic cases, including those with fatty livers.

Treating those with fatty livers by my diet, I found that, as the fatty deposits dwindled, the depleted stores of glycogen soon replenished. Except in cases of advanced cirrhosis, I found also that the diet could generally help alcoholics. Alcohol provides energy and has almost as much calorific value as fat (7 calories per gram as opposed to 9). As heavy drinkers often have little appetite, it is often the protein content of their diet which suffers; deprived of carbohydrate, they still obtain sufficient calories from alcohol. Desiring food once more, they now get enough protein as well as fat. This means that the restriction on alcohol needs be less severe for health to improve. In my view, *The Drinking Man's Diet* (Jameson & Williams, 1964) was a notable lay contribution to our medical knowledge. However, I feel a litre of beer or half a litre of wine should be the daily limit.

I did not treat viral infections of the liver with my programme, as I found that low carbohydrate nutrition can worsen their condition. However – and this surprised me at first – gall bladder patients improved noticeably on my diet and could often avoid operation. These observations led me to write an article in the *Wiener med. Wochenschrift* on pathological liver tests in relation to low carbohydrate nutrition 'Pathologische Lebertests unter Kohlenhydratarmen Diät' (1975), suggesting that the routine advising of a low fat/high carbohydrate diet for liver patients needed a rethink.

A similar tendency of values to improve on my diet was shown in those with levels of iron in the blood that were too high. Interestingly, low levels of iron in the blood also normalised on a low carbohydrate diet as I showed in my article 'Hypo- und hypersiderosen unter Kohlenhydratarmer Diät' (hypo- and hyperferraemia on a low carbohydrate diet, 1976). Blood calcium levels likewise tended to normalise on my diet, whether initially too high or too low. Now if both high and low levels of blood iron or calcium come back to normal when carbohydrate is restricted, surely this implicates carbohydrate as a possible disturber of these levels in the first place?

Right from the start I had been interested in the use of my diet for patients with heart problems. Here I was lucky in so far as the first patients I treated – and with considerable success – were all those whose cardiac insufficiency was due to excessive demands on the heart muscle, i.e. in cases for example where there were valve defects and hypertension.

When I moved on to treating patients with heart failure of unknown cause, I met with problems. Here a patient experiences difficulty with breathing and feels his heart is misbehaving; the heart is enlarged and there is fluid somewhere in the body. Normally the outlook is bleak, with the patient succumbing to his illness in a few years as, apart from heart transplants, medicine has not developed a successful treatment, nor fully understood why the heart fails.

My own feeling was that heart failure probably comes about initially through damage to the heart muscle from carbohydrate-associated catabolism, with its excess cortisol and thyroid hormones and the constant protein sacrifice needed for gluconeogenesis (for providing sugar when necessary); there may also be infection involved as well as a tendency to auto-aggression. The problems I met with when it came to treating such conditions by my low carbohydrate regime, I think came from the immune system, together with the strengthening of the growth hormone resulting from the new diet. This situation calls not just for appropriate application of immune-subduing drugs but also for diligent monitoring of immune response during the early weeks and months of the transition to the new diet.

Indeed, there are times when a doctor must face a very tricky dilemma – a sort of 'damned if you do, damned if you don't' situation, where the patient is so ill that he or she will die if you don't act immediately but might die if you do. You, yourself, know that carbohydrate reduction is the only hope for the patient, yet precisely because of the consequent strengthening of the growth hormone, there can be initial worsening before improvement sets in and therein lies the danger. There may also be unforeseen consequences.

Let me tell you about a patient of mine, who will always stay in my memory. This was an Austrian nurse who devoted her life to her calling, travelling to the Far East to inculcate paramedical methods. Eventually she reached South Africa, where her heart began to trouble her. She then came back to Austria where, going from one hospital to another, she underwent the usual treatments for oedema of the heart without success. When, at 74 years of age, she finally found her way to me (as a doctor with 'unconventional methods'), her heart was considerably enlarged and she was in a very poor way, with water retention reaching as far as her fingertips. She soon became acquainted with my low carbohydrate diet; in addition, I gave her small quantities of gold and she began to go uphill.

In fact, I was amazed at how well she did on the diet: in a few weeks she lost all the excess fluid*. She felt well again and was so happy that she offered to work unpaid in my practice, an offer I soon talked her out of. She returned contentedly to her own work and after a few months I asked her to write down exactly what she was eating – hers is the menu I included in my book *Leben ohne Brot*.

Then sadly, after six months on the diet, she died quite suddenly. Her death was thought to be due to a thrombosis with an embolism of the lung, though this was never firmly established. This patient had received dramatic help for her weak heart and water retention, but perhaps the diet had been too quickly introduced? Or perhaps she had needed protection against the formation of blood clots? I often wondered about this. This patient had experienced the joy of feeling well again for the short time left to her and at least in this I had helped her. The immune system has a long memory and cannot always learn new ways and this may have been part of the problem. I do not know.

This said, I have shown many times over, and with lasting results, that a low carbohydrate diet can prove invaluable in cardiac insufficiency. Even though not part of the usual repertoire of the cardiologist, I feel that cautiously introduced low carbohydrate nutrition should be thought of, especially when elderly patients do not respond promptly to the usual heart preparations such as digitalis, diuretics etc. It is unfortunate that the diagnosis is often made fairly late on in the condition, as I feel sure that the lives of many patients could be saved by timely instigation of the right diet.

Details both as to which types of liver, heart and other problems I thought unsuitable for treating with my diet and as to those which I found particularly responsive, are given in my articles and in recent editions of *Leben ohne Brot*.

Nutrient intake on my diet

Now to the very practical consideration of whether the amounts of the various nutrients offered by such a diet as mine were adequate. I have sometimes been asked by worried patients whether keeping to my diet would lead to vitamin deficiency in the long term. Certainly, in the four or so years during which I myself had eaten a negligible amount of plant food, I developed no detectable avitaminosis, nor had I witnessed any obvious deficiency condition – whether of vitamins, minerals or of any other essential nutrient in my long-term patients. In fact, I have seldom found the need to prescribe supplements to my patients. It seemed that patients were often better off on my diet, especially in terms of the fat-soluble vitamins A, D, E and K. I saw no rickets, for example, a condition I fear will make a real comeback with the sometimes drastic reduction of fat which people are currently making in their diet.

On my low carbohydrate diet, as long as people were eating enough meat and fat, they seemed to derive all the nutrients they needed. In saying that I had never spotted any signs of nutritional deficiency in patients who kept to the diet over a number of years, I am reminded of someone who had suffered from a lot of bowel trouble and had gained relief though upping her fat intake and reducing her carbohydrates. I first treated her at about the time of my first book and met her again a few years ago. This was the patient from whose letter I quoted in the last chapter about the difficulty of convincing people about not feeding too much sweet food to children. The letter, received in 1998, also included the following sentences:

No-one can be convinced more than I am of the correctness of your therapy, for, after seven years of torment, various useless therapies and long stays in hospital, it has restored my dignity and made it possible for me once more to live an active and fulfilling life.

You saw for yourself, when we met in Salzburg, how healthy I look after thirty years of eating à la Lutz.

E D, Vienna

As a practising doctor, you do 'see for yourself', and you have a very good sense of the overall health of your patients, especially when you see them over a period of many years. Yet, in these days of anxious 'healthy eating', I could understand the need for reassurance through actual measurements not only of vitamins but also as to, for example, the likely level of calories. I was also quite curious to find out such information for myself – if nothing else it would pacify relatives who were concerned about this!

At first, I looked for studies already done, and found that most studies looked at people who had merely switched to a low carbohydrate diet for the purposes of the study and for only two weeks or so. I found none that looked, not at the healthy, but at patients who had been recommended a low carbohydrate diet as part of their treatment and were following it over a substantial period of time. All I could do in those days was to reassure patients from my own experience as a doctor.

Later, with all this in mind, I did a study with two colleagues: Professor H Kasper of the University Hospital of Würzburg and dietician M Wild to ascertain the daily amount of various nutrients patients of mine were getting on my low carbohydrate diet, with its free choice of protein and fat. For this study (Kasper, Lutz & Wild 1979), we chose ulcerative colitis patients. The group consisted of 14 patients, 8 male, 6 female, and aged between 9 and 75 years who had been on the diet for an average of just over four years (a range of 3 months to 15 years). We chose people whom we felt were reliably sticking to the recommended diet of 6 bread units, who were in good general health and who were in remission, i.e. who were doing well and had no longer any bleeding or other symptoms (clinically obvious or shown by laboratory tests) of bowel irritation. Measurements were done over a typical week.

In terms of vitamins, the results were reassuring, showing as they did adequate intake of vitamins A, B1 and C. We did not measure other vitamins or the mineral content of the diet. But my impression is that, far from creating imbalances, the diet tends to clear up many already existing deficiencies, as already mentioned with blood iron and blood calcium levels.

In terms of carbohydrate consumption, the results were as follows: nine patients were consuming 50-100g of carbohydrate per day, i.e. roughly between 4 and 8 bread units; two people chose to eat more than this (100-140g) and none more than that; three people had chosen to eat less (40-50g). The daily average worked out at 77g of carbohydrate, of which 54% was starch, 46% sugar.

One can see that the majority of the group were in fact eating roundabout the recommended six, give or take two bread units either way. However, given we had chosen people whom we felt were reliably sticking to the recommended diet of 6 bread units, it was somewhat sobering to find that in practice the carbohydrate eaten ranged from 3 to 12 BU – so much for the supervision one can give once patients are doing their own cooking!

As to self-chosen level of carbohydrate intake, it is interesting that Robert Atkins (1994) found something similar in his work on obesity: namely that once people had satisfactorily reduced weight and subsequently found for themselves what he called the 'critical carbohydrate level for maintenance', the long-term level that kept weight stable usually ranged between 40 and 90g of carbohydrate a day.

In our study, we also measured fat and protein intake and found the average consumption of fat was 156g per day, that of protein 103g. The average fibre intake of the group was 7g daily and dietary cholesterol 750 mg. These figures implied that these patients were on average deriving 14% of their total energy from carbohydrate and 66% from fat, with an average daily calorie intake of 2,247 kcal. Note that, as one might expect, there was considerable variation of intake* of nutrients between the girl patient who was 9 years of age and the 22–year-old male patient and the 75 year-old.

It can be seen that the average daily intake of fat was higher than that of the figure for Germany (which was about 130g of fat at the time), and also that the average daily fibre intake of the group was considerably lower (German average 24g per day). To me, this latter result was hardly surprising, given these were patients who were in remission from ulcerative colitis, a condition easily aggravated by too much fibre as well as too much carbohydrate.

These patients had obviously chosen their food well, for they were all keeping free of symptoms and with a condition such as ulcerative colitis this was no mean feat. And this is the main point: the fact these patients were all doing well and feeling well meant the main aim of my diet was being achieved, i.e. to reduce carbohydrate sufficiently to alleviate their condition by eliciting a healing effect.

Further publications

Over these years, I continued to document my growing experience of this healing effect and the 1970s saw a spate of further articles covering various aspects of low carbohydrate nutrition, its boundaries, its problems and so on.

A word on Crohn's disease, a condition related to ulcerative colitis and one which I was treating more and more often. My observation was that morbus Crohn usually responded well to carbohydrate limitation. Improvement often started showing in weeks, sometimes in months, and I found no recidivism or new fistula once patients had been on the diet for a few months. I found that any early worsening lasted only a few weeks (auto-immune reactions that could be suppressed with cortisone) and the sufferer of Crohn's disease would most likely be symptom-free within one to two years, by which time blood iron would have normalised whether or not iron supplementation was given. I found that morbus Crohn responded far quicker to the diet than did ulcerative colitis, which could take many years.

And so it was that, at the end of the 1970s and throughout the 1980s, I wrote many articles on morbus Crohn, amongst others, in 1981, 'Low-carbohydrate Diet in Ulcerative Colitis and Crohn's Disease'; in 1985, 'Morbus Crohn unter kohlenhydratarmer Diät' (morbus Crohn on a low carbohydrate diet); also in 1985, 'Morbus Crohn, eine allergische Reaktion auf resorbierte Makropartikel?' (morbus Crohn, an allergic reaction to reabsorbed macroparticles?); in 1987, 'Morbus Crohn unter kohlenhydratarmer Diät, Langzeitbeobachtung an 67 Fällen' (morbus Crohn on a low carbohydrate diet, long-term observations on 67 cases).

This period of my life also saw the publication of three books. The first was a milestone in my life, as it brought my work within reach of the English-speaking world for the first time. This was my 9th edition of *Leben ohne Brot* kindly translated into English by Beatrice Idris-Duncan and Joy Wieser. It was called: *Dismantling a Myth – the Role of Fat and Carbohydrates in our Diet* and was issued in America in limited hardback edition* in 1986 by publisher Charles Thomas. The same year, my German publisher Selecta-Verlag Dr Ildar Idris GmbH & Co issued a paperback edition.

The second book, also brought out in 1986, was *Die Lutz Diät* (the Lutz Diet). It was a nicely produced hard-back book, which presented my medical work and my diet in fairly accessible form. It was subtitled: *Kerngesund und schlank endlich ohne hungern* (at last vibrantly healthy and slim without going hungry). I look back with some discomfiture at both the title and the subtitle, which I seem to remember being chosen by its publisher, for I am fully aware of both the antiquity of 'my' diet as well as its limitations.

The year 1988 saw my book *Cholesterin und Tierische Fette* (cholesterol and animal fats). The 'fat theory' was gaining ground and in this book, as in *Leben ohne Brot*, I offered not just a critique of the dubious and now all-pervasive 'fat theory', but an alternative: namely a 'carbohydrate theory', which drew on epidemiological evidence for support. In this book, I showed just how essential cholesterol is to our bodies, something not fully realised at the time.

In *Cholesterin und Tierische Fette*, I also looked at how the big American field studies* had failed to show that lowering the intake of animal fats brought about any significant decrease in the death rate from cardiovascular disease: at most, it exchanged a small drop in non-fatal coronary attacks for an increase in other diseases such as that of strokes and cancer, together with an increase in crimes of violence including suicide – a most unwelcome exchange, I would have thought.

Yes, these studies did pinpoint high blood cholesterol as a potential risk factor for heart infarcts, but FOUND NO RELATIONSHIP BETWEEN FAT AND CHOLESTEROL IN FOOD AND A HIGH CHOLESTEROL LEVEL IN THE BLOOD.

If this important distinction had been appreciated at the time, many further studies, much expenditure – and dare I say much heartache – would have been spared. Instead, erroneous and one-sided interpretations of these and other studies led Western medicine to get mired in its greatest error: that of believing that it is animal fat that makes us ill.

I wrote then that I hoped to live to see medicine free itself from its mistaken belief that cholesterol and animal fats are responsible for heart problems, arteriosclerosis etc. Yet neither I, nor those courageous others who have spoken out against uncritical acceptance of the 'fat theory', have been able to turn the tide. With all the conflicting and often unsubstantiated opinions that abounded at that time, many wrote deploring the putting forward of blanket dietary guidelines which were insufficiently backed by either reliable clinical experience or a sound and agreed scientific basis. These include Professor Hans Glatzel (1974), Professor George V Mann (1977), Professor Hermann Mohler (1978), Dr Edward H Ahrens (1979) Professor Robert Olson (1980) and Professor Michael Oliver (1983).

My compatriot Professor Hans Kaunitz fought for many years against the idea that fat has anything to do with arteriosclerosis. In the forward he kindly wrote in 1986 for *Dismantling a Myth,* the English translation of my book *Leben ohne Brot,* he said:

> Lutz'z ideas have challenged the lipid theory which also some others (like myself) believe to be built on sand . . . Lutz's approach is controversial but his ideas deserve to be tested.

Kaunitz in Lutz (1986)

His own ideas were also controversial and deserved to be tested, as from Professor Kaunitz (1978) originated the repair theory of cholesterol: namely that, in the first instance, cholesterol is deposited in places where repairs are necessary. That this repair was probably needed because of carbohydrate-induced damage to the arterial walls, both Schole and I had demonstrated with our hens.

It is some fifteen years since I wrote that book on cholesterol and animal fats and I fear that, in general, medicine is still stuck in the same fallacious – and, in terms of our long-term health, disastrous – reasoning as then. More recently, others have spoken out, including fellow doctor from Scotland, Walter Yellowlees, whom I later met and who was kind enough to include an extract from my book *Leben ohne Brot* in his own book *Doctor in the Wilderness* (1993). Yellowlees, too, was not enamoured of the fat theory and, in his book, he speaks out strongly in favour of natural fats as an essential and beneficial part of both our long-term dietary history and our present need.

My book on cholesterol and animal fats was followed in 1989 by an article 'Arteriosklerose and Krebs – Fette oder Kohlenhydrate?' (arteriosclerosis and cancer – fats or carbohydrates?), in which I again put forward my carbohydrate theory of arteriosclerosis, backed by findings of epidemiology. In it, I suggested the setting up of a study to show the favourable influence that can be achieved in coronary heart disease and other diseases of civilisation by restricting carbohydrate rather than animal fats. I felt strongly that the eating of fats according to appetite in conjunction with a low carbohydrate diet would throw a very different light on the picture. Sad to say, this call was not acted upon.

By the time this last article appeared, I was 76 years of age and still working in private practice as a consultant in internal medicine in Salzburg. Two years later, at the age of 78, I retired. However, there was so much to do in the medical line that I was soon to start up in practice again!

A Comforting Thought

Let me pick up on Professor Glatzel's phrase in the foreword quoted earlier in this chapter: 'the form of diet on which mankind lived for at least two million years*' and perhaps add 'on which we, human kind (Homo sapiens) have lived for roughly the last one hundred and fifty thousand years'. Over my long working life, which has not exactly been free from the derision of some of my fellow doctors, it has always been a comforting thought to have 'taken up' the type of nutrition that has served us and our forebears so long, for not only is it the kernel of the idea that brought the diet into my life but it gives my diet an established pedigree.

For the idea that animal-based nutrition is our natural state and that people are therefore stronger and healthier on such food is no new one, but part of our cultural tradition: one might even say it is part of our collective memory, for surely this knowledge is part of our common heritage as told in Bible stories! For instance, in the story of Cain and Abel, did not the shepherd Abel find more favour in the sight of God than his cereal-growing brother Cain?

> Now Abel was a keeper of sheep, and Cain a tiller of the ground. In the course of time Cain brought to the LORD an offering of the fruit of the ground, and Abel brought of the firstlings of his flock and of their fat portion. And the LORD had regard for Abel and his offering, but for Cain and his offering he had no regard.
>
> Genesis IV 2–5

Note that fat, the most energy efficient food and one that could be in short supply, was in those days thought of as a precious commodity and one equally appreciated in warm climates* as in cold ones. And, for anyone predisposed to equate the eating of meat with warmongering, it may be as well to remember that it was Cain, the tiller of soil who slew Abel the shepherd and not the other way around!

Did not the hunter Esau sell his birthright to his non-hunting brother Jacob for a 'mess of potage'? And do I not remember how Eve was expelled from paradise (the Paleolithic before cereals!), condemned to a future of painful childbirth as Adam tilled the soil?

> To the woman he said: 'I will greatly multiply your pain in childbearing; in pain you shall bring forth children . . .' and to Adam he said: 'Because you have listened to the voice of your wife, and have eaten of the tree of which I commanded you, you shall not eat it, cursed is the ground because of you; in toil you shall eat of it all the days of your life; thorns and thistles it shall bring forth to you; and you shall eat the plants of the field. In the sweat of your face you shall eat bread till you return to the ground . . .
>
> Genesis III, 16–19

Another account of a lost paradise is to be found in the Epic of Gilgamesh (Sanders 1972), which recounts the adventures of an ancient Mesopotamian hero, the restless and lustful Gilgamesh. In this fragmentary text, thought to be about 4,000 years old, we again meet the tensions that were coming to the fore in the Neolithic period, tensions between the ancient Paleolithic way of eating and the 'neo', i.e. new way.

And of course the tale told in the fifth century B.C. by Herodotus (III, 22), the Greek historian, is a story that I have always loved and I have told it in many of my books. It tells of the health and longevity of the Ethiopians (many of whom seemingly lived to be at least a hundred and twenty on boiled meat and milk) and of the contempt in which the new food, grain, is held by this traditionally meat-eating people, though I myself would not condemn bread as 'dung' as the King of Ethiopia did.

Incidentally, Vilhjalmur Stefansson, to whose work I devote the next chapter, was a graduate in divinity before he became an anthropologist. He explores historical attitudes to meat-based nutrition, including some biblical ones, in his fascinating book *The Fat of the Land* (1956), a book well worth a read. Like Jameson and Williams, Stefansson was another lay person who made an important contribution to medicine.

7 VILHJALMUR STEFANSSON

A hostile climate

Ever since the earth cooled down enough to allow life to flourish, there have been climate fluctuations both large and small, with cycles of heat and cold. The major characteristic of an ice age is the drop in average temperature, with a consequent expansion of the area of the globe covered by ice. When this happens, not all areas of the world are equally affected: regions near the Equator much less so than those nearer the Poles. As told in chapter 1, Europe was in the grip of the last Ice Age and already populated with small groups of Neanderthals, when we modern humans arrived here some 30 – 40,000 years ago.

By 18,000 years ago, the time when the ice sheets had spread their furthest, almost a third of the earth lay under ice up to a mile thick and temperatures in most of Europe were markedly lower than they are today: on average by about 12 degrees Fahrenheit (Chorlton 1983). Rainfall was also much reduced. Britain then was like parts of Alaska are today, and the sea around Spain was as cold as that off Greenland. In areas of Europe at the edge of the ice sheets, this meant long winters that were cold and dry, with a sudden burst of vegetation in the short summer months.

It was these climatic conditions that the Cro-Magnon encountered all those thousands of years ago, and in which they lived on the game herds that migrated between winter and summer feeding grounds, grazing on the plants in the shallow topsoil that covered the permafrost: the reindeer, wild horses, antelope, mammoths and bison. It was environmental conditions such as these, which Stefansson felt he had encountered at the beginning of the last century during his travels in the Arctic.

Stefansson in the Arctic

I would like to tell you a little more about my one-time guiding star Vilhjalmur Stefansson. At the beginning of the last century, there were a series of expeditions to the Arctic regions to study the local geography, geology, ornithology, oceanography and so on. Stefansson, who was born in 1879, was an explorer, anthropologist and ethnologist and, at first, he went along to study the local population of Inuit – or Eskimo, as they were then called – later going as expedition leader.

Thus it was that Stefansson spent a number of years travelling among the Canadian Inuit, many of whom were still living in their traditional fashion, uninfluenced by Western civilisation. Interested in learning the ways of these people, he stayed at their settlements, lived and dressed like they did, and learnt their language. Although the food eaten was very different from what he was used to, he participated in their fare. As he said himself:

> In 1906 I went to the Arctic with the food tastes and beliefs of the average American. By 1918, after 11 years an Eskimo among Eskimos, I had learned things which caused me to shed most of those beliefs*.
>
> Stefansson (1935–6)

During these trips, Stefansson noticed that the 'primitive' Inuit he encountered were very fit and well, and appeared not to suffer from the degenerative diseases of civilized peoples: they were not plagued by elevated blood pressure, coronary infarction or strokes, nor did he witness any cancer among those still eating their ancient diet. Neither did there seem to be any of our typical gynaecological complaints: he heard of no difficult births, no complications in pregnancy or problems in breast-feeding. Nor

– which particularly struck him – did he see any obesity. Stefansson knew the Inuit did not stint themselves as regards food: when enough food was available, an Inuit ate until he was satisfied. On the number of calories consumed at such times, a white man would surely have become obese, yet there was no apparent overweight amongst this people. Incidentally, it was Stefansson who first brought to my notice the thoughtful and thought-provoking work on cancer by Alexander Berglas* (1957) of the Pasteur Institute in Paris.

Stefansson was an anthropologist blessed with an enquiring mind, a combination that enabled him to grasp connections otherwise easily overlooked. Thus he was one of the first to recognize that it was not the racial origins of the Inuit that accounted for the absence of our diseases but rather their primitive form of nutrition. The traditional Inuit were hunters: they hunted and fished for their food, in some areas existing entirely upon animal matter. To me, the Inuit were the modern equivalent of the Cro-Magnon people of the last Ice Age that had set me on my own particular journey. I therefore read Stefansson's accounts of his travels with great interest.

On one of his early journeys, Stefansson stayed with the Copper Eskimo of Coronation Gulf, whom he subsequently described in his first book of polar exploration: *My Life with the Eskimo* (1913). Previous to Stefansson's visit, these Copper Eskimo had had no contact with white man and were living in every respect the equivalent of a Stone-Age existence, yet they were accustomed to take three meals a day and very often boiled their meat. (Fire, especially in the form of oil lamps for cooking and heating, was known to them long before the advent of white men with their matches!) This, I think, scotches the myth that you can only live on meat and fish alone if these are eaten raw.

Now I have heard it suggested that Europeans could not eat this way – that the reason such a one-sided diet is not harmful is because the Inuit have been eating this way a long time and so are well adapted to their diet. It is likewise easy to assume that the Inuit have a different digestive capacity from that of the average westerner. Yet no noticeable problem was reported about moving on to an all-meat diet by Stefansson who, albeit of Icelandic parentage, was a white American. Moreover, Stefansson encouraged his men to 'go native' and found that with them, too, nationality made no difference in their ability to do so, and this whether they were white European, black Cape Verde Islanders or Polynesians from the South Sea Islands.

What did present a slight barrier to change was age and customary eating habits: the younger men found it easier to make the transition to living off a diet of just fish or seal meat than did the forty-year-olds in his party. But, if there was absolutely nothing else to eat, initial squeamishness soon passed and, after a few days and within a fortnight at the most, all turned up for dinner. After six months on seal meat alone, all were willing to do the same again on future trips.

A cure for scurvy

Eating only what the land or sea provided, Stefansson felt extremely well during his physically demanding existence, travelling as he did vast distances, mostly on foot, across sea ice and tundra. During his time up North, Stefansson spent perhaps a total of nine years living on meat and water alone. (I include fish and birds under the category 'meat'.) It was long enough to experience the difference in his health that he felt when living by hunting as he went along, as opposed to living on the tinned or dried provisions generally carried by the expedition.

À propos this difference, there was an interesting incident on one of the expeditions he was leading. Early on:

> Charlie had complained of illness. On getting up suddenly, he felt dizzy and sometimes collapsed. In general he was disinclined to all exertion, depressed with all sorts of gloomy

forebodings, and his strength was noticeably less. These were the symptoms of scurvy and I asked to see his teeth and gums. The gums were swollen and purple and the teeth were slightly loose. There was a dull ache in the arch of the mouth and the gums bled readily. This was almost conclusive, but I did not see how it could be with the diet we had been having.

Stefansson (1953)

But Stefansson was no doctor: he mistook the condition for the gum disease of pyorrhoea and sent the progressively weakening man back to base with a support party, telling him that scurvy was impossible while eating fresh meat everyday.

He and three others continued with their trip on the sea ice. Two men soon began to get ill, also with lassitude, joint pains and gloomy querulousness. Again, Stefansson was puzzled until he found out that, unbeknown to him, instead of carrying out his instructions as to the daily inclusion of some fresh meat, the men had been living entirely from European groceries for several months previously. As a consequence of this, it really was scurvy that they were suffering from.

The men were unable to find seals during the excursion on the sea ice, but fortunately they had dog sleds with them to transport the two men as they got progressively weaker; the party gained land in time to kill caribou to provide the much needed fresh meat. This cured the scurvy and both men recovered their spirits and their health. Within a few weeks, both men could again walk ten miles at a time over rough and challenging ground.

When Stefansson returned from the Arctic to the USA in 1918, he wrote a paper entitled 'Observations on Three Cases of Scurvy'. This was followed, in 1921, by his second book *The Friendly Arctic*. The reaction of scientific circles to his work was both deprecatory and incredulous, appearing as these publications did in an era that was taken up with metabolic investigations and vitamins – a time when it seemed impossible that anyone could live without fresh fruit and vegetables for any length of time.

Stefansson was quite bluntly accused of publishing fiction.

Yet there was a group of doctors whose interest was aroused both by Stefansson's work on scurvy and his experience of going native. Curious to know whether his supposed and unorthodox Arctic diet had in practice done him harm or good, they suggested checking this out and Stefansson willingly subjected himself to a thorough medical going-over. To their surprise, the doctors found Stefansson – despite his many years on seal meat and caribou – to be in a state of health equal to, or better than, the average man of his age who had followed a mixed diet. This group of doctors included gastroenterologist Clarence Lieb, who wrote up the results of the 'going-over' in 1926, and Professor R. Pearl of Johns Hopkins University.

Although unable to trace any ill effects from Stefansson's stay in the Arctic, Doctor Lieb and his colleagues still had grave doubts as to whether anyone could live in modern conditions on the food of our ancestors: perhaps, on the frontier or in mid-winter, one might manage on meat and fat for awhile, but surely not an ordinary American business man, leading a sedentary life in the metropolis! The only way to get to the truth of the matter was to do a trial under strict medical supervision.

A year on meat alone

The experiment was duly set up under a prestigious committee of experts chaired by Professor Pearl, with the clinical supervision by Doctor Lieb and with the main research work headed by Doctor Eugene Dubois, medical director of the Russell Sage Institute of Pathology. It was to take place in the years 1928–29 and was, in Stefansson's words:

> to give modern science what appeared to have been the first chance in history to observe human subjects while they lived through the chill of winter and the heat of summer, for twelve months, on an exclusive meat diet.
>
> Stefansson (1935–6)

The trial, known as the Bellevue experiment, was to take place on the dietetic ward of the Bellevue Hospital in New York and Stefansson was to be joined by one of his earlier travelling companions in the Far North, a Dane called Karsten Andersen – or Charlie, as he was known. (For this was Charlie, one of the three cases of scurvy mentioned above. Once back at base camp, Charlie had been cured by Stefansson's deputy and so knew first-hand the curative value of fresh meat.)

Once he had grown accustomed to it, Charlie had thrived on the local all-meat diet. Having subsequently spent over a year without groceries, he had no qualms about joining in with the experiment. He was the more willing to participate since, in the ensuing years as an orange farmer in Florida, he had not been in the best of health. Working out-of-doors in the subtropical sunshine and on a 'normal' diet, not only did he have one head cold after another, but also his hair was beginning to fall out and he suffered from intestinal toxaemia.

Both men were admitted to the hospital and, after three weeks on a mixed diet, both started living just on fresh meat as their only solid food. According to Stefansson (1964), there now followed a period of suspense, in which leading authorities in nutrition and physiology showed 'near unanimity in the prediction of dire results': a well-respected European physiologist predicted that the two men would be unable to continue such a poisonous diet for more than 4–5 days; another eminent American physician set an outside limit of three weeks; still others expected nothing less than fatal results!

At first, both men were kept under constant surveillance: Andersen was on the ward for the first three months, but Stefansson went out under supervision. Later, both were given more freedom and Stefansson, still adhering strictly to the diet, occasionally left the city on various journeys, whereas Andersen spent the whole year in New York. The men were trusted to keep to the diet. (You can tell a lot from laboratory tests, so the doctors were quite sure that the slightest deviation in diet would be detected!)

During the 12 months of the experiment, both men were subjected to a whole battery of metabolic and other examinations. These were very thorough – anything that could be tested and measured was closely scrutinized and repeatedly examined. Few individual doctors could ever muster the resources for such intensive investigations – I was certainly never able to do so during my own working life!

What they ate

It is interesting to look at the men's choice of menu, for the two men were allowed to select what food they liked and to prepare it in whatever way they liked, as long as it came under the broad category of meat. The idea was to exclude every food from the vegetable kingdom – so no fruit, no vegetables, no batter round their fish or breadcrumbs on their Wiener schnitzel – the only exception was unsweetened black tea or coffee after a meal. Stefansson disliked coffee without sugar, so most of the time he drank water or, Inuit fashion, he partook of the broth in which the meat had been boiled.

Eggs, milk and milk products come it is true from the animal kingdom, but to avoid confusion in the interpretation of results, dairy foods were not included. (The subtext was to convince sceptical doctors of the harmlessness of flesh foods per se.) At least, they were left out of the diet as far as possible – only when there was no alternative food available, for example on journeys, did a few eggs creep on the menu. Total strictness, though, was maintained as to the avoidance of all foods of plant origin.

If you are wondering what these two men actually ate during this time, I will tell you. Basically, they ate what took their fancy: lamb chops, sirloin steak, brains fried in bacon fat, chicken, fish, liver and bacon, pork and veal. Other than the dishes traditionally served uncooked or very rare, they very seldom took their food raw; Andersen liked his meat medium cooked and Stefansson well done. Moreover, they were not given the flesh of wild animals but ate the sort of ordinary butcher's meat that you or I might buy from the supermarket. They received no vitamin supplements.

When they were able to do their own cooking, they boiled their meat Inuit-style, enjoyed chewing on the bones and drank, as I said, the cooking water. On the rare social occasion that Stefansson was to attend, he would provide ideas in advance for the baffled hostess. In fact, he even concocted a menu for just such eventualities. It started with 'hors d'oeuvre: caviar on chicken breast'!

In terms of quantity, Stefansson and Andersen ate on average 150–200g of lean meat and 50–90g meat fat at each meal. The proportion of lean to fat was left to the appetite of the men. But, despite their liberal fat intake, it turned out that their resultant calorie intake was fairly moderate: Stefansson averaged a daily total of 2,650 calories, of which 2,100 calories came from fat and 550 from protein; Andersen averaged 2,620 total calories per day, of which 2,110 were from fat and 510 were from protein. The actual amount of protein that Stefansson and Andersen ate ranged from 100–140g, fat intake ranged from 200–300g and carbohydrate intake from 5–10g per day.

On this diet, very few calories came from carbohydrate: something like 20–50 calories a day. What this means in terms of percentages, is that they derived 15–25% of their calories from protein, 75–85% from fat and a mere 1–2% from carbohydrate*. Obviously, since they were totally free to eat as much or as little as they liked, their actual intake of nutrients varied from meal to meal. (The figures I quote may vary slightly, as they are taken from different reports, the averages being taken sometimes over the year, sometimes just over a few months).

Stefansson already knew the importance of eating fat along with the lean, for he had seen how the Inuit, if they did not get enough fat and had only lean meat to eat, had soon suffered from lethargy, diarrhoea, loss of weight and general malaise, a situation he referred to as 'fat starvation'*. He knew that neither the lean nor the fat of meat provided sufficient nourishment in itself and that, when there was so little carbohydrate in the diet, it was therefore essential to eat fat as well as protein.

Nothing remarkable occurs

Thus it was that the two men continued contentedly on their all-meat diet, whilst experts watched on, anticipating serious disease or, at the very least, awaited symptoms of general nutrient deficiency. Yet, week after week went by and then month after month, and still Stefansson and Andersen showed no sign of the onset of scurvy, nor could any other sign of illness or deficiency be detected in them.

After all the adverse publicity that eating meat has received over recent years, and especially red meat with the fat left on, it will perhaps reassure readers to know that the (often daily) consumption of meat, red or otherwise, apparently had no deleterious effects on either of the men: neither then, nor afterwards according to a follow-up study done seven years later (Lieb, 1935). As far as these exhaustive tests were able to determine, the health of both men was unimpaired and their mood stayed buoyant.

Even Andersen did not sicken, as might have been expected by those who believe meat harmful for the gut: instead, he felt very well indeed. Shortly after he went on the meat diet, he noticed a 'marked decrease in the shedding' of his hair though, like mine during my own guinea pig years, the balding patches did not grow new hair. During the entire year, he had but one or two head colds. What is more, Andersen completely lost his former intestinal complaints, which had worried him in Florida when he was on a so-called 'normal' diet and could have all the fruit he could eat.

The results of the experiment were subsequently published

in great detail: see for example Tolstoi (1929), Lieb (1929), McClellan and Dubois, (1930), Torey and Montu (1931). There were a great many reports on all aspects of the findings, from bowel flora to kidney function and bone density. I can mention only a few of these here, for they would fill the rest of this book!

Interestingly, stools tended to be smaller and less frequent on an all-meat diet, as was noted in the traditional Inuit. According to Dr Lieb (1935), the Bellevue meat diet caused a simplification of the intestinal flora and a marked reduction both in types and total number of bacteria. Torrey and Montu (1931) wrote that the faeces of both men had 'an inoffensive odor and [were] entirely unsuggestive of putrefaction'. In neither man was there evidence either of digestive malfunction or of gaseous distension.

As to weight, Andersen weighed 60kg at the start of the trial and 58kg at the finish. His blood pressure before the diet was 140 over 80 and, after the year on meat, 120 over 80, whereas Stefansson's blood pressure stayed constant all year at 105 systolic and 70 diastolic. Neither of them showed ill effects on their kidneys, on their circulatory systems or on their cholesterol level. Stefansson's cholesterol reading was 263 mg per cc before the diet, 315 at the start and 212 mg per cc after a whole year on meat and fat.

Both men were taking only as much exercise as expected of a normal New York businessman. Yet in neither was there a decrease in mental or physical vigour. If anything, in Stefansson, physical stamina increased as the period of dieting progressed, even though he led a very sedentary year, writing and lecturing.

There was no evidence of reduced blood calcium levels in either of them, and their teeth did not decay; their gums showed no sign of pyrrhoea and no bone loss could be detected. Meat is said to be stimulating, but there was no striking elevation of metabolic rate in either of them. In fact, at the end of the experimental year, the comment made by Dubois was that: "the most remarkable thing about the experiment was that nothing remarkable occurred." For me, this very absence of any 'remarkable' occurrence is, in itself, significant. For what better indication of the suitability of a type of food than for the body to stay contentedly within its normal operational boundaries – or, as with Andersen's body, that it even improves in health?

Here I am reminded of an old gentleman that I met some years ago. I had given a lecture on my dietary ideas and afterwards a 75–year-old man approached me, saying that he agreed with my ideas since they matched his own observations: his hale and healthy wife (then 88 years of age) had never yet had a day's illness in her life. It turned out that his wife's father had been a game-keeper on a large estate and the family had been free to eat as much game as they liked; his wife had consequently eaten nothing but meat as a child and had grown so accustomed to it that she had kept up the habit throughout her life!

To live on meat alone was, admittedly, an unusual choice in 20th century Austria. But, as regards the eating of meat, fashions change. Stefansson recalled how, in the 1930's, it was of lean meat that many Americans were afraid, believing animal protein to cause hardening of the arteries and high blood pressure. He noted how times had then changed and fat was avoided and lean meat praised. But the pull of carbohydrate as part of 'civilised living' is strong and, when the Bellevue experiment was over, Stef went back to the standard American diet with its substantial proportion of carbohydrate, a decision he was later to regret.

Stefansson's return to his 'friendly Arctic' diet

Now Stefansson hoped that his time on meat would set him up and protect him from the ills of the 'white man's diet'. Perhaps it did to some extent: it may have postponed for a few years, or lessened the severity of, the stroke he was to suffer in 1952 at the age of 73. One cannot know.

I only came across the work of Vilhjalmur Stefansson

towards the end of his life and had no chance of making his acquaintance personally, though I remember sending him a manuscript of something he wanted. In his reply, after thanking me Stef complained that, since it was no longer produced in the USA (because of the fat theory he knew to be false), he had to travel all the way to Canada just to obtain his beloved liver sausage!

By the time of his letter to me, having had physiotherapy and drug treatment, Stef had again taken up a regimen similar to that followed during the Bellevue experiment. When I heard of his death in the summer of 1962, I wrote to his wife Evelyn, who told me how, with his return to what he called his 'friendly Arctic diet' (after the title of one of his books) Stef had become calmer and more at peace with himself, and how he had adhered to the meat diet for some six or so years until his death at the age of 82.

For the last few years of his life, Stefansson had been working on his autobiography *Discovery*, from which I quote below. This was published posthumously in 1964, with Evelyn adding a postlude. In it, Stef documents how the improvement he had experienced on changing his diet enabled him to get back to his writing. In the final year of his life, he wrote:

> I [now] work at my typewriter about twelve hours a day – perhaps half that on Sundays . . . Samples of my blood have been taken . . . It is enough to say that the results have been contrary to the accepted theory. Blood pressure dropped when I transferred from a mixed diet to a diet high in fat. The cholesterol count also dropped with the long-continued use of a large intake of hard fats, chiefly mutton and some beef . . .
>
> As to how it seemed to me when at seventy-six I changed from the helter-skelter mixed diet to the present one, it seemed that I became ten or twenty years younger. Except for the results of my stroke noticeably chiefly in my right hand, my joints are still behaving themselves about as I remember them twenty years ago. Pain disappeared from

all joints after a few months of high fat diet. It has not returned. My hip joints, which used to awaken me several times a night have not disturbed me since 1955.

Stefansson (1964)

Though my own hip trouble had come much sooner in life than his, Stefansson's account of his joint troubles and consequent change of diet resonated with my own early experience, even down to the disappearance of hip pain and the relief and rejuvenation I had felt as the burden of pain and soreness lifted from me and I was able to return to an active life again.

An all meat diet is something that many people would find difficult even to imagine and it is certainly something I have never personally requested, even from myself. Yet, having seen how safe and how helpful an all meat diet can be, I hope the reader will be somewhat reassured that meat in itself qualifies as a sound basis for a long-term diet. I hope, too, that the reader will have fewer qualms as to nutrient intake when contemplating my own more mixed diet, especially patients who for the sake of an irritated gut might have to eschew fruit and vegetables for a while to facilitate their own healing.

8   LATER YEARS

Our heritage

Right from the start, shall we say of my deviation from the strictly orthodox, I had been interested in the fact that some countries seemed to have more than their fair share of the 'diseases of civilisation', and wondering whether and how this might be linked to carbohydrate consumption. Looking to epidemiology for clues and remembering how, historically, agriculture had radiated outwards from Asia Minor I attempted to correlate the incidence of modern disease with the time factor of this spread. I argued that the seeming preponderance of our modern diseases in the northwest as compared with the southeast might possibly be explained by the much shorter period these countries had known grain, giving them less time to adapt to increased carbohydrate consumption than those European countries which had known cereals longer. I published an article to this effect in *Medical Hypothesis* called 'The Colonisation of Europe and our Western Diseases' (1995).

We still do not know enough about the level of carbohydrate the body can handle efficiently without compromising health too much, nor how much this varies between individuals or even between populations. There are many, many unanswered questions! Has any level of physiological adaptation to an increased level of carbohydrate taken place? Would some degree of adaptation explain, say, the variation in the response of my chickens? Do differences in carbohydrate tolerance show in our genes? Was Stefansson right when he suggested all those years ago that the inertia of the genetic makeup of a higher animal (including man) was such that the few thousand years during which man has practised agriculture, and the couple of hundred that have elapsed since he discovered how to produce sugar, were far too short a time for any noticeable effects to have taken place? (To me, this idea of insufficient adaptation had always been a ray of hope: the light at the end of the tunnel through which I had to pass, whilst working in a medical environment hostile to my notions of diet.)

Judging by the skewed distribution of various diseases, some nations did appear to cope better with carbohydrate than others; on the other hand, surely the genetic material of a baby entering the world today is remarkably similar to that of its ancestors of 20 – 30,000 years ago, who decorated their caves with paintings and supported themselves almost entirely by hunting game? If so, the implications are that we have the teeth, the nervous system, the hormonal system and the digestive system, and therefore the same dietary requirements, not of some previous species such as those of a great ape, but of man, the hunter, man, the scavenger, man who occasionally supplements his need for food with roots, shoots, leaves and fruits in season.

In 1998, I went to Oxford to meet Bryan Sykes, professor of genetics at the Institute of Molecular Biology, whose work is tending to confirm this immediacy of biological family.

> . . . each of us carries a message from our ancestors in every cell of our body. It is in our DNA, the genetic material that is handed down from generation to generation. . . It is the traveller from an antique land who lives within us all. . . the history of our species, Homo sapiens, is recorded in the genes that trace our ancestry back into the deep past . . . These genes tell a story which begins over a hundred thousand years ago . . .
>
> Sykes (2001)

Professor Sykes and his team were working on genetic sequencing, including genetic mutations, tracing the ancestry of different groups of people right back in time. In his very readable and fascinating book *The Seven Daughters of Eve*, which came out a few years later, Bryan Sykes identifies seven clusters – the daughters of Eve – of identical genetic sequences. He claims that virtually all Europeans are descended from these seven 'daughters'.

The extensive DNA sampling that Sykes and his team carried out into mitochondrial DNA indicates that the ancestry of the great majority – at least four out of five – of modern Europeans can be traced back directly to six of these 'daughters', who lived in the Upper Paleolithic period before the advent of agriculture. (Mitochondria are the tiny energy producing 'factories' that are found throughout the trillions of cells in our bodies; mitochondrial DNA is passed on by mothers to their children, giving instructions on energy production.) Now, to my mind, surely those of us who, in terms of our energy metabolism, are the same flesh and blood, as it were, as the Cro-Magnon of the last Ice Age, have inherited a metabolism designed to derive its energy, not primarily from carbohydrate foods, but largely from dietary protein and fat?

There was, however, a seventh 'daughter'. Discussing my ideas, I found that Sykes, too, was interested in the spread of farming from the Near East that has taken place in Europe since the last Ice Age, though from a different viewpoint. Geographically, he found the location of the genetic descendents of the migrating agriculturalists (the farmers of the Neolithic who cultivated cereals and domesticated their livestock) to coincide almost exactly with the two main routes taken by the early farmers (as confirmed by archaeologists) one into central Europe, the other along the coast of the Mediterranean, along the Spanish and Portuguese coasts and up to the west of Britain. Interestingly, the gene sequences of these descendents could be not only traced back to this one daughter but also to no more than 10,000 years ago, i.e. no further than the beginning of farming.

Energy production is necessarily related to food intake. In terms of the seeming variability in our susceptibility to various carbohydrate-induced modern diseases, I feel it therefore may prove relevant from which daughter of Eve we are descended. But I am no geneticist and whether the differences that have been distinguished between the mitochondrial DNA of the descendents of the farmers (with their more recent genetic sequences) and that of the majority of Europeans who seemingly descend directly from their forebears in the Ice Age sheds light on any difference in tolerance of carbohydrate, I must leave to others to determine. Nevertheless, we are reminded that, subtle differences apart, the design of our energy system is not only a remnant of a bygone age but also – and crucially – the system by which we still operate today. Maybe, as I have long contended, this is the crux of the matter!

My American book

By this time I was in my eighties and, after my very temporary retirement, I was again busy with my patients. I was also still writing. The year 1995 saw the publication of a slim volume of mine, which concentrated on the help a low carbohydrate diet can offer towards alleviating diseases of the intestinal tract; it was called *Kranker Magen, kranker Darm – Was wirklich hilft* (ailing stomach, ailing bowel – what really helps). It covered the whole gamut of gastrointestinal ailments, including the rectification of disturbed stomach acid regulation, stomach and duodenal ulcers, polyps, chronic diarrhoea, gastritis, diverticulosis, constipation and cancer, as well as the already mentioned morbus Crohn and ulcerative colitis.

I continued pursuing my medical work in Salzburg. However, things were changing in my life and, at the age of eighty-two, I had the good fortune to marry again. My new wife, Helen, an Austrian by birth, had been accustomed to live in London and I therefore began to spend more time in England myself. This I am still doing, in fact we are both now enjoying spending our winters in England and our summers in Austria.

In order to be able to practice whilst in England, I registered with the British Medical Association. This was in 1997 at the age of 84. My particular intention was to help people with gastrointestinal disorders, and especially the many with Crohn's disease, an area that has recently claimed much of my attention as a physician. Dividing my time between Austria and England did mean new patients, of course; it also helped me be accessible to patients in both countries. In this way, I could still keep in contact with patients, when necessary over a long period of time – something which, as a physician, I feel to be important.

As I get older, my book *Leben ohne Brot* gets fuller. I remember many a time producing new material at the very last minute, hoping it could still be squeezed in: it usually has been, thanks to Dr Idris and her patience with me as an author. This book, into which I have poured any new insights or findings, was to become the main repository of my observations and ideas. In a way, it tells my story better than any autobiography can do. Each edition offers the next episodes of my discoveries in treatments, setbacks, the ideas of my contemporaries and my own continual theorising, and this in addition to the evolutionary theory and rationale for my basic diet, which the original 1967 edition contained. Later editions have a more extensive carbohydrate table and, by request, a fortnight's menu plan and recipes. *Leben ohne Brot* has been continuously in print for forty or so years; it is currently in its fourteenth edition, with a new edition planned and still selling!

My translation of its 9th edition: *Dismantling a Myth – the Role of Fat and Carbohydrates in our Diet* was by now long out of print and so, to facilitate my work in the United Kingdom, in 1998 I issued a 30-page summary of Leben ohne Brot in English. Sometime before then, I had met in Washington an American biochemist, Christian Allan, who then came to visit me in Salzburg. Chris was very excited about my ideas, including those on cancer, and he asked my permission to use my material to write a joint article together with a Russian scientist who was working in the field. This I willingly gave and looked forward to the result though, sadly, it came to nothing,

Chris Allan and I thought of finding a publisher to reissue *Dismantling a Myth* in America but to no avail. Chris then proposed that he and I should write a new joint book on low carbohydrate nutrition, based on *Leben ohne Brot*. I was delighted by the idea of interest from an American publisher, and hence of my work being spread further amongst English-speaking peoples. As *Dismantling a Myth* was in any case somewhat out of date, I arranged for parts that had been recently added to *Leben ohne Brot* to be translated* from my 14th German edition for Chris to work on and include in the new book.

The book *Life without Bread: How a Low-Carbohydrate Diet Can Save Your Life* eventually came out in the year 2000 – my personal contribution to mark the millennium! I was proud to have made the American scene once more: it was a special day and the end of a paragraph in my life. My own health was quite frail that year – I was 87 by then - and I did not go over to America for its inauguration as I had hoped. Nor did it quite take the world by storm as I had also hoped!

A doctor is firstly responsible to his patients, so I am unhappy about the frequent use of 'we' in the medical sections, as in 'we have found in these cases medium doses of cortisone . . .'*. Had Allan, who is Doctor Allan by virtue of his Ph.D., put: 'I, as a layperson, have also observed . . .' it would have read less as though Allan and I were both doctors of medicine. I also feel that more on precautions could have been included with advantage and was sorry that, through pressure of time, I was not personally able to make these adjustments.

On the whole, though, I was pleased with the book and have been glad to receive letters of enquiry about my work as a result. I am happy to report that my ideas on cancer* were included and so did get an airing in the English language this way. *Life without Bread* was first published by Keats, which has since been taken over by publishers McGraw-Hill. The book has now been translated into Polish. It is good to have an outpost in America and hope that Chris Allan will continue to promote my work for many years to come.

Colleagues

By the time the American book came out in 2000, I had had more than forty years of relevant experience – long enough to be sure in my own mind of the value of low carbohydrate nutrition both as a long-term prophylactic diet for the healthy and in the treatment of many diseases. That year, I had the pleasure of meeting Dr Jan Kwasniewski from Poland, who wrote *Die optimale Ernährung* (Optimal Nutrition) in 1999. In Jan Kwasniewski, I found a fellow spirit, who also saw in erroneous diet the vast morbidity of the Western world and who, like me, used carbohydrate restriction as the appropriate healing tool for many of today's ailments.

How many of us there are in this field of the therapeutic use of low carbohydrate nutrition, it is impossible to know. I have frequently met young doctors in the German-speaking world who practise my methods, but who choose to do so without publicising the fact. But I do know that we 'old stagers' with long experience, who have spoken out in our books, all had our own notions as to what a low carbohydrate diet meant and our pet formulas* as to how to translate this into practical advice for our patients!

Here I am thinking of doctors like Blake Donaldson and Robert Atkins, as well as myself and Jan Kwasniewski. All four of us saw the natural food of man as being predominantly that of food from the animal kingdom, food that fulfils our basic need for protein and fat. We shared, too, the basic tenet that food should be as suitable as possible for the human metabolism and that the best and most efficient fuel for the body to run on being fat, together with a small amount of glucose. We all claimed to treat many of the usual diseases of civilisation with some degree of success.

Given the prevailing consensus against animal fat, it is worthy of note that both Donaldson and Atkins started out as heart specialists (as also did Pennington); moreover they continued to treat heart problems using a low carbohydrate, fat rich diet. As my speciality was internal medicine, heart problems also came within my brief, as already told. All of us witnessed the reduction of excessive cholesterol in many patients fed on a so-called 'high cholesterol diet'. Jan Kwasniewski claimed that intermittent claudication (a cramp-like condition of the legs often caused by atherosclerosis) could to some extent be reversed by his diet. I myself admired the fact that he had the pluck to treat it: namely, atherosclerosis was a condition I was merely hoping to prevent!

Apart from its general suitability to our whole metabolism, we four doctors likewise had our favourite focus for explaining the basic mechanism by which our diet worked. For Atkins it was weight loss through ketosis and, for me, the rebalancing of the hormonal system by a return to our ancient diet. For Kwasniewski, it was rebalancing the functioning of the autonomic nervous system and for Donaldson in *Strong Medicine* (1963): 'Everything goes back or rather forward to enough amino acids in food'*.

However, whatever we thought the underlying mechanism, surely the most striking thing was that we were all, I think, in accord that, on our own respective diets (which all, in their own way, restricted carbohydrate, allowed protein but by no means restricted hard animal fats), there tended to take place in our respective patients a noticeable level of repair and regeneration.

A diet for life

Like consultation, correspondence with patients is a necessary part of my medical life and a lot of my time is still involved with this. In 2001, after publication of my American book, I received the following letter:

Dear Dr Lutz,

Thank you for your recent letter. . . . I so deeply appreciate what you have done in writing your books to try to help people in ill health, and to take your own time in following up with us is so touching!

I have been on the diet religiously . . . [for] almost 3 months now. It was difficult at first, since I am used to (and prefer) eating almost entirely carbohydrates. It has gotten easier, and I have seen some improvement, however am struggling with a few adjustments. As I'm sure you're aware, a limit of 72 grams of carbohydrate daily also severely limits calories . . . . . . I have lost weight I didn't want to lose. I was about 119lbs. to begin with, and am down to about 109, which is a bit thin for me. Also, I am constantly exhausted, which I am guessing is from weight loss and reduced calorie intake . . . I realize this will be a long road to getting well, but I remain committed to the diet, expecting to be on it for at least a year . . .

I Y, USA

I cannot comment on this particular case (medication and a bowel problem were involved here), but I include this letter to show how people could get the wrong end of the stick and hence how difficult it is to get a message across in a book or by letter.

I had, I thought, been clear that the thin often initially lose weight. Moreover, I am not aware that my diet 'severely limits calories': indeed, I do not place any limitation on calories (with the occasional exception of the severely obese, where short-term calorie cutting was needed to achieve the desired weight reduction). Nor have I ever pretended that mine is a diet to get people well and then to be abandoned: after eating 'almost entirely carbohydrates', the change was a big one and it could take months and maybe much longer to adjust to the new diet and, in so far as carbohydrate caused or aggravated the medical problem in the first place, my diet has to be seen as a way of eating for the long term – better still for life!

Books are all very well but, in my experience, there is no

substitute for personal consultation! You see, sometimes, even patients who have become and ostensibly stayed well on the diet may begin to worry and become anxious and so need personal advice and reassurance. Here is a letter I received in 2002:

> Dear Dr Lutz,
> . . . about twenty years ago, through your low carbohydrate diet you helped me avoid the removal of part of my colon or worse. In those days, I came to your practice from deepest East Friesland, suffering from a blooming ulcerative colitis. Then I turned up at intervals of 2–3 years and you could yourself witness the quality of life I regained through you. My last severe relapse is now 10 years ago. Anyway, it was the first since your first treatment, and I have followed the diet ever since . . .
>
> R O, Rhauderfehn

The above letter goes on to ask whether, despite bad hospital experiences before she came to me and despite 10 years without relapse, it was time to go back to hospital for a new check-up 'just in case'. Others want purely to communicate a success story, as in the following letter I got in the year 2000.

> Dear Dr Lutz,
> . . . In 1996, I phoned you. At that time, an operation had been advised because of a conglomerate tumour in Crohn's disease. I then chose not to undergo the operation. I also stopped the medication. Since then, I have been fine. I have kept to the low carbohydrate diet and enjoy the best of health.
>
> My life has moved on in leaps and bounds. I married, achieved my doctorate and have had two daughters and got a job as scientific assistant at a university. I can't say how helpful the diet has been in all this – surely without it all this would not have been possible! I am now trying to publicise low carbohydrate nutrition for Crohn's patients and, of course, your book . . .
>
> K O., Koblenz

Still other letters are accompanied by a full clinical update, as was the following note of personal gratitude from an old patient of mine, written in 1999 at the age of 74 years.

> Dear Dr Lutz.
> I am writing on the 25th anniversary of my 'Lutz diet'. A diabetic for 27 years, I have been on your diet for 25 and have coped very well through all stages of my illness . . .
> When I consulted you in 1974, you told me I could get by without medication and so it was. I was soon labelled stubborn in my circle, as I never allowed myself to be led away from the straight and narrow under any circumstance. To this day, I weigh my bread, my potatoes and so on, using diabetic scales . . .
> It was only in 1990, when I suffered from some severe attacks of fever and had to take antibiotics, that I could get by no longer just with your diet . . . I must say, that when having to stay in hospital for various short periods, I always succeeded in talking the dieticians into letting me carry on with your diet.
> I owe it to your diet, Dr Lutz, that I managed for 16 years without medication and even today need only low doses of insulin in addition.
> I remain gratefully yours,
>
> S M, Salzburg

Naturally, problems crop up and there are issues to be discussed, especially when people have been self-treating. There can be many ideas – such as that the body might react differently to different carbohydrates – that are new to them and the significance of which they might need help in grasping. For instance, in 1997, I received a letter from someone suffering from morbus Crohn who tried my diet after reading my book, who writes:

> My condition got significantly better and meantime I feel almost normal. However, if I eat only one piece of bread
> . . .
>
> M H from Gänsedorf

When patients complain of getting their symptoms back, say diarrhoea, when they start putting a particular source of carbohydrate back in their diet, I suggest to them that, since it was probably carbohydrates that made them ill, perhaps their body was telling them something: in this case, that 'only one piece of bread' is one piece too many! My advice is simple: to avoid eating bread and possibly other flour products, and to try other (to them more tolerable) carbohydrate sources instead such as potato. There are some people who may be sensitive to the fraction of wheat called gliadin (gluten), if so they would also need to avoid anything made from gliadin-containing cereals (wheat, oats, barley and rye) to see if this helps.

Finally, I would like to quote an extract from 'Report on my illness: ulcerative colitis / morbus Crohn, and their healing', written to help fellow sufferers by Renate Paulitschko (her real name) of Gersthofen.

> I was born in 1951 and suffered for 8 years from ulcerative colitis, an inflammatory bowel disease with ulceration. As I have been healed since 1985, I have a need to write about the course of my illness and my cure. My only wish is to help other sufferers, for only those who suffer from Crohn's or ulcerative colitis can know what it means to be confronted with this illness for the rest of one's life. One knows from personal experience that that there is no cure, at least from the doctors and medical scientists. According to the medical profession, this condition is incurable, and therefore attempts are made at alleviation. This means continual investigations of the most unpleasant sort, continual visits to the doctor, laboratory tests and much more, not to mention the pain, the loss of blood, the discharge of foul-smelling mucous, circulatory disturbances, depression, tiredness, flatness, weakness, the continual urge to defecate and much more. My own case shows that all this does not have to be so, as do the hundreds of cases of a doctor of internal medicine named Dr Wolfgang Lutz from Salzburg (address given).

In 1984, I read in a journal an article by this doctor, who claimed to heal this disease with a simple primitive diet . . . Treatment lasts between 1 and 8 years, according to the severity of the condition; with most people 1–2 years . . .

In January 1984, I therefore started with the diet and with great success! After eight years [of suffering], the first ray of light! Gradually, all symptoms grew less acute . . . I felt newborn and there awoke in me the lost ability to take pleasure in life. It was May 1984 before I was free of trouble and showed no or almost no blood loss.

Certainly, my bowel was regenerating, but had not healed. I knew this because if I sinned by eating sweets and esp. pastries, I experienced an immediate relapse. This proved to me that the illness was completely connected to the false nutrition of our generation. For if I kept strictly to my low carbohydrate diet, my condition really did improve again within a few days . . .

Moreover, in order to avoid relapses, the diet itself is to be practised for life. For the body will surely be susceptible for life, I think . . .

Dr Lutz has been fighting for 20 years to at last conquer this illness, investing time and money, and not least his energy. I find that amazing, especially as this great doctor is not acknowledged by medicine and science. Perhaps because he achieves success without drug treatment. I do not know . . .

Paulitschko, 1986

I do not know either! And it is true that recognition has been hard to come by: I remember going from town to town, university to university, in an attempt to get together enough interest to do proper scientific trials on Crohn's disease. It is not enough having hundreds of grateful patients – you have to prove your therapy by particular methods, for instance by what is called a prospective randomised trial.

It was a long time – it only happened in my later years, in fact – before with the help of Frau Dr Erdmuthe Idris I got such a trial on its feet: namely Crohn's Study V. It was a proud moment for me when the results showed significant and enduring results from carbohydrate restriction (Lorenz-Meyer, 1996). However, honour and recognition did not follow – despite my efforts in convening the trial, I was not even acknowledged in the write-up!

Nor, in my opinion, did they reduce the carbohydrate low enough to show what my diet really can do for this illness. This was because, although I had instigated the trial, I did not personally supervise the patients, whose carbohydrate intake was only reduced to 12 – 13 bread units. Nevertheless, as I said, the resultant improvement in the trial patients with Crohn's disease was held to be statistically significant, which in itself is interesting. Note that merely reducing sugar had not achieved this result, but only the restriction of total carbohydrate, something I have always felt to be important.

Nowadays there is much talk about the quality of fat and especially about unsaturated fatty acids such as omega-3, said to have certain metabolic effects. I do not doubt these scientific assertions but I doubt their clinical importance: for we compared the results of putting Crohn's patients on my low carbohydrate diet with those to whom we gave omega-3 without reducing carbohydrates: omega-3 appeared to have no effect on those taking it, whilst those on my low carbohydrate diet improved.

My own health in later years

I was, as it were, the first patient whom I treated with a low carbohydrate diet. As I shared my medical condition at the time of my conversion to this form of nutrition and told of my early days on the diet, the reader will expect an unadorned account of my subsequent medical history. I also give this at the specific request of some of my patients, for instance:

> Dear Dr Lutz,
> You have helped me a lot with your book *Life without Bread*.
> I would have been in a wheelchair long ago had I not changed my nutrition.

I have even been to visit you in your practice with my wife so that we could be personally instructed . . .

It would interest me extremely to know your own health in your own old age. I am perhaps 10 years younger than you (1922) and feel healthy and capable of work.

With good wishes from your book reader and patient,

D I-O, Waltersburg

This was written in 1999, when I was 86 and the writer a mere 77 years old!

So how am I in my 'old age', and how have I fared in the intervening years? The reader knows how, after my 'conversion', I led an active life once again and that I had no more migraines, no corns, no dental caries, and I soon became able once again to work full tilt and after a while was able to return to my sporting hobbies. But what about my subsequent 'half a life without bread', as I like to call it?

Well, I proceeded to have twenty almost trouble-free years, during which time I again played a lot of tennis and enjoyed my time on the ski slopes. The freedom to do this was wonderful, but perhaps I overdid my sporting activities, as my left hip eventually needed replacing. This was when I was 65. In the same year, I developed persistent sciatica during a transatlantic flight and needed a lumbar fusion. I was told then that it would not be long before my right hip, too, would need replacing! Yet I remember at 72 being able to compete in sport with men far younger than myself.

In fact, my right hip served me well for a further twenty years. Then, after contracting Lymes disease (the aftermath of a tick bite, which I received whilst walking in the woods near my home in Austria), my right hip became very painful and I doubt whether I will get back to how I was before the tick bite. By then I was in my late 80's, an age at which a hip operation carries a certain risk, so perhaps I will get by permanently with my old one! I also suffered from another ruptured lumbar disc, but have not needed another orthopaedic operation.

Obviously the diet, though it had restored my mobility and banished the pain for so many years, had not cured my arthritis per se. Perhaps one cannot expect a restructuring of the joints through a reshaping of bones deformed by arthritis? Interestingly, all these years later my X-rays still show the same bony changes and reduction in cartilage as they had done previously in the 1950s. Yet, except for the formation of cysts at the femoral head, there has been little further degeneration in all the intervening years.

However, even if they do not regain their shape, I am convinced that bones strengthen on my diet. I recall taking my wife to a ball in a London hotel a year or two ago, when I had the misfortune to tumble down a whole flight of marble steps. I was taken to hospital for a check-up: I was a bit bruised but, to their surprise, no bone was found to be broken. I remember my wife commenting that she admired the strength of my bones, but that she could have done without me putting them to the test in this way! So as not to give a misleading impression, I must add that my ribs were not proof against a fall that happened the year before against the rim of our bathtub!

Looking back, I ask myself where the arthritis came from in the first place. Well, I remember that, as student at Innsbruck when I was in my twenties, I had had several bad falls on the icy ski slopes of the Tyrol and the damage done during these mishaps probably contributed to the development of my arthritis in the first place. I said earlier that my hip pain had started about eight years before I began the diet. Thinking about it, I remember having X-rays on my hips in my thirties, whilst in the internment camp, so my hips must have been troubling me even then, my left one in particular: perhaps it was also to do with malnourishment in the camps.

Whether my left hip only held out because of certain periods of laxity around that time as to 'counting the carbos', or whether it was because my advancing years made it more difficult for my body to cope with the anatomical changes in my hip joint,

I do not know. Nevertheless, I think I owe to the diet the fact that the hip operation, which in 1957 had seemed so imminently necessary, had been delayed for so many years. At the time, I was comforted by the thought that I had probably brought it on myself by playing too much tennis!

If I had my time over again, I would be kinder to my joints and lumbar discs and put less stress on them once damaged and I would certainly avoid eating so many carbohydrates (in my student days I had a great love of sugar and sweet foods). Then, without a constant call on my insulin, my growth hormone would have ensured a better tissue quality and therefore I would have been more robust in health in my youth and my skiing accidents might not have led to such detrimental consequences. Likewise with the wearing down of my lumbar discs: I did not know then of the deleterious effect of carbohydrates on connective tissue or this, too, could have been avoided.

Yet, though the arthritic aftermath of my skiing accidents (together with that from years of carbohydrate overindulgence) proved less reversible than I had hoped, I did, as I said, experience a lot of improvement in mobility and strength and, mercifully, not just the alleviation but the absence of pain in walking and in sports over a great many years. All things considered, I am grateful that my joints have lasted so well for so long.

The family burden

I have been asked about my disappointments as to the effect of my diet on my own health. Obviously, one issue was my inability to go for brisk walks in my old age because of the eventual return of my hip problems. The other main disappointment was that I did not entirely escape the family burden of high blood pressure, high uric acid levels and, alas, arteriosclerosis. I realize that it is a particular irony that, I, as a pioneer of low carbohydrate nutrition, should suffer from these things. Indeed, I hoped our ancient diet would shield me, but it was not so. To some extent I was already troubled by them in my sixties, if not before, and they have been part of my lot for a great many years now.

Looking back you realize how early the seeds of future trouble are sown and how the first signs are often making their appearance without you paying much attention at the time. Take arteriosclerosis: in the prison camp I already suffered from dizzy spells, so the problem may well have been present even whilst I was still in my 30's, and well before I started on my carbohydrate-reduced diet. Much to my regret, a scan, done later during investigation of my hip problems in my 60's, showed some signs of arteriosclerosis* in my major arteries.

Much later still, at 86 years of age, I had an unpleasant reminder in the form of a slight stroke. This was in the autumn of 1999; I myself was aware only of a slight dizziness following two glasses of wine. There was no paralysis, but my brain was a little affected: it seemed that my stroke had resulted from an embolus, which left a tiny part of my brain without sufficient blood supply. On analysis, the surrounding tissue showed traces of arteriosclerosis, as I saw on the slides done at the hospital in Salzburg. However, after a small operation on my left carotid artery, things are a lot better. In fact, I recovered fairly fast and according to the last investigations, the affected artery now functions well and the blood flows smoothly again. My thinking is also a little clearer – well, I think so!

So what have I got to say about uric acid? Well, here is a curious thing. I measured the uric acid level in the blood of a group of my patients in response to carbohydrate restriction; 4 out of 5 of my patients responded favourably to the diet and their uric acid level went down. It was a good result and worth people knowing about, but I remember the displeasure I felt when the success rate was not the 10 out of 10 that I had hoped for! In respect of uric acid, it seems that I am one of the minority who do not respond favourably. With my brother, it is the same, so perhaps this is partly a familial gift from my grandparents?

It was likewise with raised blood pressure: I found that, in the majority of my patients, high blood pressure responded well to carbohydrate restriction and tended to drop, just as the level of uric acid had done. Yet, as with uric acid levels, not all cases of high blood pressure did so: a minority, especially those patients whose levels were particularly high to start with, required medication in addition to the diet to achieve this reduction. Given my family history, it would be surprising if I were not part of the few who eventually required the intervention of drugs.

Here one must also remember that some types of medication for treating high blood pressure can in themselves cause a rise in uric acid levels. I do wonder if this, in itself, may increase arteriosclerosis in patients being treated in this way? I wonder, too, if I could have avoided both my hip operation and my tiny stroke had I controlled my uric acid levels during the second half of my life through appropriate medication? Perhaps so, I do not know.

As to raised blood pressure, in my case I feel that congestion in my hip joints may have something to do with it, for I have noticed that prolonged sitting aggravates it and a brisk half hour walk used to relieve my blood pressure considerably – unfortunately, a type of exercise I can no longer enjoy. A diet, free of any salt except that which occurs naturally in food, is an extra measure I have adopted in recent years with some degree of success.

How far heredity – the family burden – played a part in my high blood pressure and so on, it is difficult to gage. On my mother's side of the family, there have been many instances of high blood pressure, strokes and heart infarcts: my maternal grandparents both died of heart attacks between sixty and seventy years of age; my mother's brother died of a heart attack in his fifties and my mother's sister died of a stroke, so I was from a family already plagued by the diseases of civilization.

All in all and for whatever reason, in my old age, I have not turned out quite the shining example I had hoped to be for the diet I advocate! But you see, maybe I am a bit like those of my hens that reduced their carbohydrates after a third of their life on a high carbohydrate feed, and who did not fare as well as those birds which were fed on a low carbohydrate feed from soon after birth. Except for the fact that I had spent not a third but half my life on a potentially damaging diet, perhaps I was like my chickens in that my change of diet came too late to prevent at least some changes in my blood vessels?

On the positive side, these same chickens suffered less than their peers who did not cut down on grain. So, despite my nearly 45 years on a high carbohydrate diet and my inherited predisposition to these medical conditions, maybe my low carbohydrate diet has exerted some protective effect. Certainly I feel that my blood vessels have profited from the change of diet and seem to have achieved a reasonable tissue quality. So far, unlike many of my family, I have only had the one minor stroke and am still here to tell the tale.

In terms of predisposing hereditary factors, my prospects certainly seemed gloomy. However, I took heart from the fact that my great-grandfather (the one with the mill) achieved a fair age before dying of a stroke and my father, who lived for the rest of his life in rural Austria, also stayed in relatively good health. In fact, he reached his hundredth year before succumbing to heart failure! I therefore retain a certain optimism about reaching a grand old age, as I always put my father's long life down to his eating a lot of meat and fat when he was out on his visits to his farming patients!

And my cholesterol level?

Now here is another curious thing: despite forty-five years on a diet in which I take 70% or more of my calories from hard animal fats, my current reading for so-called 'bad' cholesterol is very low. Now this is the very opposite result from that expected by the adherents of the fat theory on two counts: firstly a low cholesterol count did not in itself guarantee me complete immunity from trouble with my arteries, which according to the fat theory it is supposed to; secondly they believe that eating animal fat puts up cholesterol levels, which in me it has not done – and I have many long-term patients, who have also shown lowered cholesterol and other blood fat values after spending decades on my diet. Interesting is it not?

Cholesterol	164 mg/dl
Triglycerides	66 mg/dl
HDL – Cholesterol	61 mg/dl
LDL – Cholesterol	90 mg/dl
Qchol/HDL	2,7

Figure 8.1: Lipid status of Dr Lutz at 90, read on 12.09.2003

total lipids	847mg%
neutral fats	288mg%
total cholestero	251mg%
free cholesterol	89mg%
ester cholesterol	162mg%
phospholipids	7. 8mg%
iodine count of lipids	78
cholesterol quotient	1.29

Figure 8.2: Blood lipid values taken on 20.2.1961, after approx. three years on a grain-free, minimal carbohydrate diet (Lutz 1962)

In Figure 8.1, you can see the result of the test, which was done this autumn. Over forty years ago, my total cholesterol reading was already down to 251 mg /% after three years on my diet, as you can see in Figure 8.2. Note that by the time I had spent a full 45 years on a low carbohydrate, high fat diet, the reading shows a further reduction of total cholesterol to 164 mg /%.

(Please note that one cannot compare all the readings because of the different methods of recording used nowadays.)

In summary, having eaten according to the principles set out in this book for most of the second half of my life, apart from not entirely escaping the 'family burden' or the long-term consequences of early injury, I have been in good general health the whole time.

Taking a long view, I am sure the diet has helped me not only grow stronger and more resilient but keep so. After all, at 44 years of age, I was struggling to get through a day's work yet, by reducing my carbohydrate intake, I experienced an impressive increase in my mental and physical capacity: after that, I worked pretty well non-stop for the next forty-six years! Moreover, on the diet, I also enjoyed an appreciable improvement in my general well-being and mood, which I feel has been sustained over the years. What lies before me I cannot know but, at 90 years of age, though not in the peak of health, I am still writing, still reading medical journals and I am sporadically still seeing patients. I am also still travelling, still driving my car and still enjoying an active social life, not to mention the occasional glass of whisky!

My diet in old age

This brings me to my next topic: my diet nowadays. Since I described in detail what I ate in my 'guinea pig' years, I feel I should mention what I am eating all these years later. After my initial trial, I soon upped my carbohydrate intake and since then have been having nearer six bread units than the former two to three plus alcohol. Now that I am living without salt, the plate of cold cuts of meat that I used to enjoy for supper with my glass of beer is off the menu. In essence, though, my diet is no different now, but to satisfy the curiosity of the reader, I will be specific. Obviously my routine varies to be hospitable to visitors, but when we have no guests, my daily fare is more or less as follows.

Breakfast is simply a strong cup of espresso coffee from dark-roasted Ethiopian coffee beans, accompanied by single cream (18% animal fat).

For lunch, I might have a cutlet of lamb or pork, or some spare ribs cooked in butter. I am also partial to beef consommé with egg and, in winter, homemade vegetable soup. With my meal, I will sometimes have lager with 4–5% alcohol. For desert, there may be some grapes or an orange or – now and then – a small pudding or ice cream.

For my evening meal, I will again have meat, much as I did at lunchtime: just lamb or pork chops, possibly duck or occasionally a goulash; alternatively, I may have some fish or white cheese. To follow, I may take a small banana or dessert such as a crème caramel or a Florentine biscuit, and a glass of beer.

And yes, I admit to a partiality for whisky during the day and in the evening it has been known for me to indulge in the occasional 'After Eight' chocolate when watching television! So, as you see, my own 'Paleolithic diet' has been very modernized, and I still pamper, albeit very modestly, the sweet tooth I have never quite lost. As I get older, I find I take less sugar in general and, in fact, never took much since going on the diet – you cannot do so with a carbohydrate limit of 60 – 70g!

I have such a longstanding habit of avoiding starchy food that I hardly ever take pasta, rice or potatoes with any meal, though when eating out I might occasionally indulge in a small bread roll. For cooking, I use butter or the fat that comes with the meat – when I can get it, that is – and sometimes we use olive oil. Except in the delicious soup my wife cooks me, I seldom eat cooked vegetables but, with a meat meal, I often enjoy a green salad or I may take a glass of fresh vegetable juice.

Quite probably I will be criticized for eating sugar (which some people are best totally avoiding, as I mentioned in an earlier chapter). My own opinion has always been that, barring special circumstances such as already discussed in chapter 5, as long as you keep the carbohydrates low enough, it does not much matter in which form you take them. Anyway, I do not proffer this personal information as an example for people to follow: on my diet, individuals must make their own choice of what to eat – whether to eat a little bread or to exclude it, and likewise with vegetables, fruit, alcohol or coffee.

It is the same when we come to the issue of breakfast: though I frequently urge my patients not to omit breakfast (especially initially until their bodies have got used to the new routine), except for my coffee and cream, I myself prefer to go without breakfast. With me, after all the years that I have spent on my own diet, any trace of false hunger is a thing of the distant past and it suits me well to postpone eating until later in the day.

Future plans

Letters and phone calls that begin: 'I know you are retired but may I still come and consult you', make me smile. Two years ago, for example, I received the following letter:

Dear Dr Lutz,
Last year I phoned you about my ulcerative colitis of 10–year standing . . . you were kind enough to offer me a consultation despite your advanced years. Since I have been virtually bread-free for about 10 months, I am doing really well, as has been confirmed by recent [internal] investigations . . . after this success, I would, if possible, like to consult you again.

Two co-patients, one male and one female, whom I knew formerly and who are also doing well after reducing the bread in their diet, would appreciate coming with me to see you.

D V, Horb-Dettingen

That was in 2001 and I am still receiving similar mail. So, even though my health problems have slowed me down quite a lot, I still do what I can to help those that wish to consult me. How can I refuse?

I still do a lot of reading, trying to keep up with what is happening in medicine and, at the moment, I have an important project in mind: namely when I am back in England again this winter, I hope to interest colleagues in a research project on heart failure. So many old people succumb to this deadly disease on the loving pharmaceutical care of their doctors that I wish to demonstrate the therapeutic possibilities of low carbohydrate nutrition.

Stefansson's autobiography was his last work. Whether this current book of mine, which has more autobiography in it than any of my previous ones, will be my own swan song I do not know. Certainly, if not books, I am still planning articles. You see, our knowledge on the relationship between carbohydrates and sex hormones is far from complete. History tells us that, in the Neolithic, increased fertility and increased pregnancies accompanied the transition to a carbohydrate-rich diet. I know from my own work that the carbohydrates in our diet are apt to exert profound effects on sex hormones, especially by raising the levels of oestrogen secretion. Might it not therefore be possible that too high an intake of carbohydrate could lead to an exaggerated and even unnatural sexuality? Be that as it may, there is one article in particular, which I would like to get out soon, and this concerns carbohydrate intake in relation to female problems.

Remember how my low carbohydrate chickens exhibited the egg-laying pattern of wild birds? Well, when their reproductive days were naturally over (in terms of their lifespan) and their ovaries were now no longer required, we found that they shut down, whereas the birds fed a high carbohydrate diet still had active ovaries at the end of their third year. My theory is that, when women experience grave problems with what is popularly called 'the change', something similar is happening: namely an inability to shut down easily and naturally a function that is now no longer appropriate.

In my article, I hope to explore the hormonal scenario that

I think lies behind this and will try to show a problem menopause is in fact the end result of a whole chain of events that is kick-started by eating a level of carbohydrate that constantly elicits increased insulin secretion. The secretory cells of the Islets of Langerhans then grow in number and/or enlarge to cope with the extra demand and there sometimes develops a tendency to overproduce insulin, even for it to get fixed in overproduction. Increased insulin secretion in turn affects all the other major endocrine hormones: it demands more and more compensatory measures, not only from the endocrine glands (and so increased pituitary activity, thyroid and adrenal) but even from the cells themselves, that is until this is no longer possible.

You then get the phenomenon of insulin resistance* and other system breakdowns; illness ensues, not just female problems, but the whole gamut of modern diseases from diabetes to heart failure and more. However, when looking for a remedy, it is easy to make the mistake of targeting later links in the chain, which can complicate matters and may induce further problems (as for example giving hormone replacement therapy for menopausal problems and so increasing the risk of cancer). Diabetes, together with its complications, is a late stage of carbohydrate overload; the early stages are far more insidious and seldom recognised for what they are. To really tackle manifestation of multiple disturbance, in so far as it is still possible to make any real difference, one has to go right back to the original root, i.e. where the problems stem from in the first place – the carbohydrate effect brought about by excess carbohydrate consumption!

Salt, too?

I am also turning over in my mind a book about the possibly dire effects of adding salt to our food. This is another aspect of diet, which has always worried me. Here, I am thinking in particular of cancer. I was reminded of this idea by a comment made by Dr Albert Schweitzer in his Preface to the book on cancer by Berglas (1957). Schweitzer, on arriving in Lambarene* in the Gabon in 1913, saw no cases of cancer amongst the indigenous population. This was in the equatorial jungle two hundred miles from the sea. Yet, over the succeeding forty years he witnessed the gradual appearance and increasing incidence of cancer, and this Schweitzer attributed to the introduction of the foods of white Europeans, and in particular to the introduction into their diet of salt.

For me, this idea was 'grist to my mill', for it fitted with the scenario of my 'back to the conditions at the beginning of life on earth' as one explanation of cancer*. You see, our genome (the sum of our genes) forgets nothing: in other words, we have a memory inside us that extends back to the early days of life on earth, days in which bacteria-like single undifferentiated cells lived and multiplied in the primordial ocean, which was rich both in carbohydrate and in salt but with little oxygen content. My theory, at its simplest, is that if we flood our bodies with glucose through the overconsumption of carbohydrate, our bodies (from the cells' point of view) come to resemble conditions like those in the days of the unicellular organisms.

In this situation, some cells become – and start behaving like – primitive (undifferentiated) cells once more: they take their nourishment mainly from carbohydrate and tend to ferment rather than respire (which needs oxygen); these cells, though still part of the human body, are no longer subordinate to the higher organism and so can multiply recklessly. Cancer cells which, for whatever reason, have become primitive again (the process of dedifferentiation) may well find in this 'primordial soup' a favourable milieu in which to feed and divide, and surely the more so with added salt? If so, just by sufficiently restricting carbohydrate, might we not deprive our cancer cells of their basis for living, or possibly by just restricting salt? However, surely it is better to consume a minimum amount of both?

I mentioned earlier that Schole and his colleagues had shown that a low carbohydrate diet reduced the incidence of cancer in experimental animals when challenged by a known carcinogen (Schole et al., 1978). I mentioned, too, my own impression as to this matter, based on observation of my patients, and signalled the importance of maintaining strong immune function (through not unnecessarily depressing the growth hormone by too much call on the hormone insulin). Insulin resistance nowadays is increasingly seen as a risk factor for this disease; not only that, but the big field studies showed that a low fat, low cholesterol, high carbohydrate diet led to a dramatic rise in the incidence of cancer, so perhaps time will prove me correct in my suppositions. Meanwhile, I can only offer my thoughts and my limited experiences to add to the on-going debate on this topic. Conclusive evidence I must leave to others equipped to do the appropriate research.

On a more personal note, my own mother died of cancer, as did many of my relatives on my father's side. I have now lived on a low carbohydrate, low salt diet for 45 years (salt-free for the last two or three) so, hopefully, I shouldn't contract cancer myself* – at least if my theory is correct!

À propos my last comment, a sad reflection: that is that my good friend Jürgen Schole, who did such wonderful work on the subject, did contract cancer. When, in the final stages, he was already bed-ridden and without hope, I went to bid him farewell. Jürgen looked up into my face with an expression of knowing and rueful irony that I'll never forget, and then said very quietly: "I didn't do the diet, did I!"

With all this in mind, I have again been looking at the history of our relationship to salt from the very earliest days, this time from the viewpoint of hormonal regulation. We do need some salt, of course, but I have long suspected that excessive salt intake – like other excess – forces the body's regulators to make such efforts to cope (both directly and indirectly) that we eventually sicken – and here I am not thinking of cancer but of our health problems in general.

So let us leap from the unicellular organisms in the primordial ocean to the time when there were fish swimming in our seas. Fish could obtain the oxygen they needed from the seawater they swallowed and they could easily dispose of the carbon dioxide by way of their gills. Salt was freely available. Creatures, as they emerged from the ocean (whether as amphibians or reptiles or to become dry land animals) needed a mechanism to provide this exchange between oxygen and carbon dioxide: hence the development of lungs. Animals living on dry land also needed a mechanism to conserve salt and to oversee the salt and water balance in their bodies. Hence the development of the renin-aldosterone chain, an adrenal based regulatory hormonal chain that is still retained in modern humans.

Our Ice-Age diet, being predominantly of animal food, contained enough salt for our physiological needs, just as it contained enough carbohydrate – or perhaps I should say, provided the wherewithal to manufacture enough carbohydrate – to ensure a stable supply of blood sugar. It is more or less this level of carbohydrate and salt intake to which, in my view, our hormonal organisation is still geared and which it routinely expects.

We humans have, I fear, moved very far from our original diet. Over the millennia, in respect of both carbohydrate and salt, we have moved from frugality to abundance, often to overabundance. It is the opposite situation to that for which these regulatory hormones originally evolved. Our regulators still try and maintain equilibrium but, instead of having conservation and recycling as primary tasks, they are now called on to prioritise the disposal of excess; instead of husbanding scarce resources, they work overtime trying to mitigate the potential damage threatened by overload.

Such a change of emphasis inevitably has its costs: capacity for fine-tuning may be damaged, sometimes to the extent of the failure of the regulatory mechanism itself. In the case of too high a carbohydrate intake, we have seen how insulin, in response to threats that compromise the stability of the blood sugar, has to sanction obesity* and how excessive demand on the insulin-producing beta-cells of the pancreas can eventually lead to their exhaustion, that is to diabetes and a rise of sugar in the blood. Thus, the very regulatory measures necessary to deal with this situation of surplus can lead to the most unwanted circumstances that are not conducive to health.

May it not be likewise in the case of our modern habit of habitually adding salt to our food? You see, in ordinary circumstances, our salt-retaining chain is activated in emergency situations such as might occur in famine or after serious injury: namely in cases of hypotension, blood loss, excessive loss of sodium or water, and its net effect is to raise the blood pressure to a safe level again. I cannot help wondering whether a situation demanding constant hyperactivity of this system (hyperaldosteronism), such as the unrestricted use of salt in food preparation, may, through damage to that system, lead to the raising of the blood pressure to a pathological level?

Excessive salt is harmful in other ways, too. We know that it leaches calcium from the bones and we are all aware of the trouble our old people have with osteoporosis. Moreover, the chalk which has been dissolved from the bones is brought to the kidneys to excrete, and may be deposited there as chalk-containing kidney stones and on the teeth as plaque – surely another reason not to use the salt cellar without thinking, either when dining out or when cooking at home?

I am glad to say that the call nowadays is for the general population to reduce both sugar and salt, and this is to be lauded. However, to my mind, the call needs to be, not just for us to cut down on salt and sugar, but rather for a very modest intake of total carbohydrate of any kind and from any source. We also need to recognise that energy has to come from somewhere and to stop demonising animal fats. It is all too easy when 'cutting carbohydrates' to not replace the missing calories with fat, but to try and eat more protein instead, which is not to be recommended.

All in all, perhaps the best prophylaxis against the development of many of our diseases of civilisation is, as I have long been suggesting, a return to something akin to our Ice-Age diet – and by 'akin' I mean slightly more liberal – that is, we should allow the free partaking of food from the animal kingdom, including the fat, together with some additional food from the world of plants with a limit placed on carbohydrate. In other words, in my view, the best preventative treatment would be to follow the sort of dietary guidelines I have been advocating in this book and, indeed, have been doing for the last forty-five years. It is a way of eating which, after all, has the longest pedigree of any diet in human history!

I am an avid reader of the magazine *Nature* and other publications. My old interests retain their fascination for me and I have again been reading up on creatures that, like primitive fish, pertain to our early development. One such is the coelacanth; this ancient ancestor of terrestrial vertebrates, as you might know, exemplifies the time of transition between ocean dwelling and adaptations to life on land, and so possesses primitive lungs as well as gills – but that is another story!

As for hobbies, I do have a few: that is apart from ancient history and epidemiology. Remember my great-grandfather, the one who built the improved model of the mill he saw in Paris and who was always inventing things? I think I must have inherited something from him, for I enjoyed designing my own house in Hallwang, outside Salzburg. Even in my old age, I am still designing engines and still applying for patents. In fact, I have several patent applications in at the moment. One is for a new type of piston action for a combustion engine.

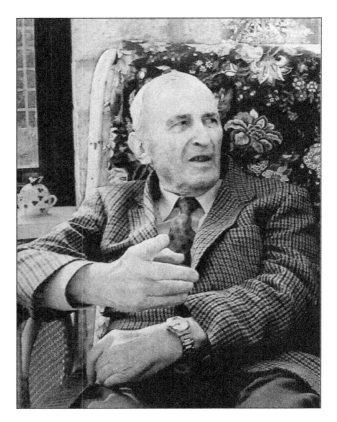

Figure 8.3: Wolfgang Lutz at 90   Photo by Monica Groves

The 27th May of this year, 2003, saw my ninetieth birthday and I was duly fêted at my London club, the Athenaeum. It was a fine affair, including a meal with toasts and speeches. One of the guests was Barry Groves, a friend and fellow enthusiast of low carbohydrate nutrition, whose wife Monica took the above photo of me at 90, when Helen and I visited them at their home. At the end of his speech, Barry kindly asked the gathering to salute my 'valuable contribution to the science of health'. This I sincerely hope I have made. I personally do not need salutes and praise, but I am only too happy when my medical work is given recognition.

In June, we returned to my native Austria as planned. In July, we moved from the Salzburg area to take up residence in Graz in southern Austria, where from now on we shall spend our summers. We hope to leave Austria again in early October before the snows, as my wife and I still plan to return each autumn to 'over-winter' in the milder climate of England – a pattern we enjoy.

I now bring this short book to its conclusion with a question and answer session.

9   A TOOL FOR HEALING

Patient Talk

This chapter comprises an informal discussion on my work, in which I answer questions asked by my patients, especially by those who are just embarking on my diet and are new to low carbohydrate nutrition either as a therapeutic tool or for general well-being. Sometimes I am asked such questions by phone or in writing as, previously, I always gave my address and phone number at the end of my books. Here, however, I feel it might be helpful to discuss my diet in the chatty informal way I might do in my consulting room, when face-to-face with a patient.

I had my own investigative equipment at my practice and, naturally, any necessary diagnostic procedures will have already taken place. I will therefore have a fair idea as to what is wrong with the person sitting opposite me. I will have decided that a change of diet is appropriate for their particular illness and I will have explained to the patient what this involves in their case. After this, there are so many questions that come up again and again that I would like to go through some of the most frequent ones here. In practice, I would try and tailor the answer to the patient concerned but, obviously, in print I can only answer in a very general way,

It is inevitable that I repeat myself to some extent in this chapter, as all topics mentioned here are covered elsewhere, most in this book, some in my other books. Please note that reading the following discussion is not a substitute for reading the whole of this book: especially chapters 4 and 5 in which the detailed application of my diet and the modifications and cautions necessary in particular circumstances are discussed.

When I first discuss food as an essential part of treatment, I always do my best to reassure my patients about the content of the diet that I propose. Before coming to see me, many have learnt that they should base their food choices on carbohydrate, with some protein and a minimum of fat. In fact, many of my patients are actually worried about the prospect of eating fat, and especially animal fat. Given the myths that surround this topic, this is perhaps not surprising, and so it is with this 'old chestnut' that we will start our question and answer cum discussion session.

The question of fat

Q: Dr Lutz, if I stay on your diet, does this mean I will be eating too much fat?

Dr Lutz: Not at all. Once you are established on the diet, you will eat only as much fat as your body is comfortable with; this may be a little more than you used to eat or it may even be a little less than formerly. One reason for this is that you will probably find you eat less commercially prepared dishes, so there will now be few hidden fats. On this diet, your own body will protect you from eating too much fat – you will soon feel nauseous if you try to!

This protective reaction seems to be more effective once carbohydrates are restricted, so a lot that you hear about the perils of eating too much fat does not apply, especially once you have been on my diet for a good while.

Q: But Dr Lutz, isn't fat high in calories?

Dr Lutz: Yes, and that is precisely why you won't need such a tremendous amount of it – a little goes a long way! When you've been on the diet awhile, your digestion will be more efficient and you may well find yourself choosing to eat fewer calories than before and feeling the more energetic for it.

Q: But, Dr Lutz, should I force myself to eat fat?

Dr Lutz: Again, not at all. If you force yourself your mind will object to the diet, even if your body doesn't – which of course comes to the same thing. No, if you take things slowly and easily, then you will find that, as you get accustomed to eating less starch and sugar, i.e. less carbohydrate, you will be able to eat enough fat for your needs and no more.

Adding fat can make food tastier. Eventually, you may well find that you enjoy the culinary delights this can bring, but this might take time.

Q: So I won't put on extra weight by eating butter and cream?

Dr Lutz: You might, especially if you need to. Weight loss is a big topic. However, you may well be happily surprised that cutting down carbohydrate in favour of such treats as fresh whipped cream on your coffee, may well reduce your weight and help you keep it normal.

Q: I am just a stone overweight. Would I lose it?

Dr Lutz: Again, you might. If you have been suffering from fluid retention then you will probably lose some superfluous weight initially. After that, what you have to bear in mind is that fat is very light, whereas muscle is heavy. On this diet, you may lose surplus water and surplus fat, but you are likely to gain sturdier bones and muscles. So, if you are not too overweight to start with, you might end up the same weight as before, but healthier for it and with a better figure, which of course is an added bonus.

Q: It seems odd to me. Surely eating fat makes you fat?

Dr Lutz: Not in itself. Let me put it this way: eat lots of fat and lots of carbohydrate and you will probably get obese; eat lots of fat and very little carbohydrate and you probably won't.

You see, fat can only make you fat if you are also eating a lot of sugary and starchy food. When we eat a lot of carbohydrate of any sort, the blood stream receives a lot of sugar, of which it can only safely carry a certain amount at any one time. The body can store very little carbohydrate; a small quantity can be converted into glycogen, a sort of starch for emergency use by the liver and muscles, but most of it has to be changed into fat.

If you eat little carbohydrate, then any fat eaten can be used by the body either straight away to make energy or else stored and easily retrieved for the same purpose, and without making us obese. This can also be true of eating a medium amount. But eat too much carbohydrate too often and this body fat is not easily retrieved to make energy, as the body then prioritises the storage of fat over its use. Obviously, if you go on eating too much carbohydrate, the fat stores can pile up.

Q: But, Dr Lutz, I have a friend who lives on cake and biscuits and soft drinks and is as thin as a rake.

Dr Lutz: That, you see, is the other way that an excessive intake of carbohydrate is dealt with by the body: it is 'burnt up', as it were, and a lot of energy is released, often leading to hyperactivity. Also food is shunted pretty fast through the alimentary canal. Both ways involve elevated levels of insulin as well as of cortisol and the thyroid hormones T^3 and T^4, but I have never fully understood why some people veer to the anabolic and some to the catabolic side of the resulting imbalance. Certainly both types of response seem accompanied by diminished tissue quality. All this will no doubt be elucidated one day.

I expect your friend is what one calls a 'live wire'? People like that are usually restless and 'always on the go' – that is until they eventually 'burn out' and get ill or chronically tired.

Q: Dr Lutz, can your diet help someone who is too thin?

Dr Lutz: Indeed it can, but the process is not always straightforward, as some people may lose a little more weight at first. With time, though, they gradually become sturdier and their faces fill out. After awhile, their figures and weight normalise. I have known it many times. In fact, I would specifically recommend my diet as a treatment for the over-thin.

Q: Why do you think this is?

Dr Lutz: I think it is basically to do with the calming down of both the nervous and hormonal systems, which tends to happen with my diet. Eating a balance of food, which is more normal in the sense of nearer to our original diet as humans, has a normalising and balancing effect on the body processes. People then cease to 'burn themselves up' with so-called nervous energy.

Q: We are told that hydrogenated fats are bad for health. Would you agree?

Dr Lutz: The fact that highly processed fats may be damaging to our health goes without saying. I would always advise the use of traditional fats that have been a long time in our diet and have not been too denatured by man.

Q: So, Dr Lutz, is yours a high-fat diet?

Dr Lutz: Only if you reckon on the proportion of energy you will get from fat – a difficult thing to do at the breakfast table! All this business of 'high fat' and 'low fat' leads people astray. Nowadays, these words are emotive but not necessarily meaningful. Eat all so-called low fat foods and you can easily have too little fat* to maintain good health.

No, the actual amount you will choose to eat when on my

diet will vary according to the level of activity you engage in, even according to your age and size, and will probably vary from day to day and meal to meal. Your appetite for it will be your guide.

Cholesterol

Q: Will this diet put up my cholesterol level, Dr Lutz?

Dr Lutz: Another old chestnut! The short answer is no, the diet is unlikely to put up your cholesterol; on the contrary, it will probably lower it, especially if your cholesterol level is high and you are young enough. But in any case, the diet is likely to make the cholesterol count less significant as a so-called risk factor.

Q: I have heard that cholesterol is vital to the health of our cells. If your diet lowers cholesterol, might it not lower it too much?

Dr Lutz: It is true that, yes, enough cholesterol is vital to our health. But rest assured that no, the diet, in itself, will not lower the level of cholesterol past where it is meant to be. I have had patients who have been decades on my diet, whose cholesterol level not only reduced but also stayed low, yet always within the range of what is considered normal. I have never once observed a fall of cholesterol below normal values from merely following my diet.

The artificial lowering of cholesterol levels through drugs is another matter. Certainly, one should be wary of medicated foods such as so-called 'cholesterol-lowering' margarines. I do not include them in my dietary recommendations.

Q: But won't eating cholesterol-containing foods damage my arteries?

Dr Lutz: Personally, I am convinced that it is not the eating of animal fat but the eating of carbohydrate that causes both our blood cholesterol to rise and our arteries to clog. Judging by my observations, if the intake of carbohydrate is sufficiently low, arteries are not likely to be damaged by eating cholesterol-containing foods, or any type of animal fat for that matter. My chicken feeding trials showed a significant reduction in arteriosclerosis when fed a low (or even a medium) amount of carbohydrate compared to high carbohydrate feed.

I am against sudden transitions but, once you are well-established on the diet and so are eating a minimum of carbohydrate, eating saturated and other fats is, I think, both safe and desirable. However, it is possible that eating a good deal of fat when one is also over-eating carbohydrate may prove a different matter – even then, it may still be that carbohydrate is the main culprit in any arterial damage, with fat proving an agent of repair.

Q: Does your diet have some sort of magic action then, Dr Lutz?

Dr Lutz: Not at all, at bottom it is as simple as this: eating my diet, you are eating a diet that is more compatible with the healthy functioning of the body than a diet that is excessively high in carbohydrate. On my diet, the body tends to produce a more favourable level of the growth hormone and hence a general improvement of the tissue quality*, including that of the arteries.

Q: But Dr Lutz, can so many people be wrong about it being bad for you to eat food containing cholesterol?

Dr Lutz: Sometimes there is a borderline between truth and error which, once crossed, cannot easily be crossed back again but rather leads to ever more compounding of the error. There was a very large field study in the USA, which started in 1948, called the Framingham Heart Study; the results highlighted blood cholesterol that was too elevated as a risk factor for heart attacks and this was well publicised, whereas played down were the Study's findings that too low a blood cholesterol posed a risk for cancer, strokes and violence.

Importantly, in normal individuals (that is those who do not suffer from high cholesterol as a hereditary condition), no correlation was shown between dietary cholesterol and elevated blood cholesterol (Gordon, 1971). In other words, this study failed to show any connection between eating cholesterol–containing foods and high cholesterol in the blood, yet this finding was, shall we say, conveniently overlooked and a myth was born, a myth which has been growing in size ever since until it has become an entrenched belief almost beyond question.

There was an eye-opening article by G V Mann 'Diet Heart, End of an Era', written in 1977. Mann, a doctor of internal medicine like myself, was also a nutritional biochemist who was an associate director of the Framingham Study for three years. You see, as Mann points out, it has not just been politics, science, education and medicine that, intentionally or otherwise, have perpetuated the myth – there have also been powerful commercial enterprises involved whose interests lay in veiling the truth.

Calmer nerves

Q: Will eating less carbohydrate calm my nerves?

Dr Lutz: Well, I myself became much less irritable once I started out on my 'Paleolithic' experiment! Others have found a similar improvement in their temperament and I have had many letters testifying to the comparative peace of mind patients have experienced since going on the diet. Restored calm is certainly one of the things found by many patients well established on the diet.

Q: You say the diet calms you down. Why do you think so?

Dr Lutz: In my view, much of the nervous tension of our Western civilization comes from the overconsumption of carbohydrates: amongst other things, from the resultant raised level of cortisol and other 'fight and flight' hormones, which is one of the body's responses to increased insulin production. This makes people excitable and agitated and they sleep less well. In hormonal terms, it is a sort of constant 'emergency action' to deal with an unwanted situation – in this case an unnatural balance of food intake.

When, by reducing carbohydrates this action is no longer called for, the regulators, both hormonal and neural, revert to their normal everyday tasks and peace descends. The peace probably comes from the mood leveling effect of the stabilizing of the blood sugar level and of the consequent calming of the thyroid and adrenal glands: that is from a more balanced hormonal situation.

But, for whatever reason, my diet seems to restore order and therefore to promote unprecedented calm to various systems of the body, including the nervous system. Perhaps this restoration of metabolic equilibrium is behind the substantial help my diet offers to ailments such as new cases of multiple sclerosis and certain types of epilepsy*?

Q: So will the diet make me a nicer person?

Dr Lutz: That I cannot say! Of course, a diet cannot change one's intrinsic character: a quick-tempered man will still retain his tendency to temper, but he may be sparked less easily. Likewise, someone liable to mood swings may find themselves more buoyant and their moods more even.

I am reminded of an amusing misprint in the book: *Eat Fat and Grow Slim*, written by Richard Mackarness. After talking about the contribution of American doctors to the field, he was kind enough to include me: 'to show that there are good European doctors thinking and working along the same lines.' He quotes 'some convincing personal testimony to the efficacy of a low carbohydrate, free calorie diet' from my book *Lieben ohne Brot*, which translates not as '*Life without Bread*' but as '*Loving without Bread*'!

Perhaps in terms of the benefits of this diet to mood and consequently to geniality, there is some hint of truth in this slip of the typesetter?

Q: Will I be able to concentrate better?

Dr Lutz: You may well discover a renewed ability to concentrate, to think at leisure or even just to stay awake after meals. I remember my co-writer Chris Allan commenting that those students who had participated in trying out the diet no longer felt sleepy after meals and so no longer fell asleep in his afternoon lectures!

Q: So would hyperactivity in children respond to your diet, Dr Lutz?

Dr Lutz: As I said, the diet seems to have a profoundly calming effect on the nerves and a normalising effect on the hormonal system, so yes, I would expect it to have some effect on hyperactivity as it works to calm both the body and the mind.

It might also be necessary to avoid various provocative foodstuffs, such as certain food additives and things they are allergic* to. I have little experience in this field, but some adult patients report that, after following the diet for a while, they are less sensitive to certain foods than formerly.

Q: Dr Lutz, might Alzheimer's benefit from carbohydrate restriction?

Dr Lutz: Dementia is a failure of the brain's intellectual capacities and morbus Alzheimer, which is associated with continual loss of memory function, used to be an infrequent form of this. Recently, the incidence of Alzheimer's has increased alarming. Old people, especially, suffer from fear of this mental derangement because harmless disturbances of memory often accompany ageing.

In so far as this illness is closely related to arteriosclerosis*, my own view is that it, too, will probably prove connected to carbohydrate overload. But this I must leave others to demonstrate.

Fewer infections

Q: Is it true that cutting down carbohydrates can reduce the number of infections one catches?

Dr Lutz: This is certainly my own experience and that of many of my patients.

Q: Will I catch fewer colds? And if so, why?

Dr Lutz: Very probably, for a diet too high in carbohydrate seems to affect the efficiency of the immune system. The wholesome balance of the endocrine system can get disturbed by such a diet: namely, the continual demand for high levels of insulin in the bloodstream elicits a high level of cortisol, both of which are antagonistic to the amount of growth hormone necessary for good immune function.

What this means is that, on a diet consisting of too much starchy or sugary food, individuals will be less able to resist infection. However, on my diet, you may still catch one occasionally, of course.

Are carbohydrates bad for us?

Q: I thought carbohydrates are supposed to be good for us!

Dr Lutz: Don't get me wrong. Carbohydrates are an integral and useful part of our food. When eaten in moderation, they can to some extent substitute for eating fat, for if not required as sugar, the body can easily convert them into fat, its preferred main energy supply. The key here is 'when eaten in moderation', for then the body can access this fat.

Q: What is wrong with getting most of our energy from carbohydrates?

Dr Lutz: There are several problems with getting most of our energy from carbohydrates, including the way our energy metabolism is set up to derive most of its energy from fat. You see, there is only so much energy that the body can usefully make from carbohydrate. Most of what can't be 'burned up' immediately has to be stored as fat which, if a lot of carbohydrate is eaten, can lead to obesity.

You have to remember that the human body, though very sophisticated and very adaptable, evolved at a time when nothing was handed to you on a plate – and especially not food! It was a hard physical life of frugality with only occasional plenty; conservation was essential and our regulatory hormonal system was therefore equipped to oversee recycling activities and the storage of every spare morsel of animal food that could be obtained. (Carbohydrate from plants would have been minimal and seasonal, if present at all.)

Nowadays, this situation has been reversed: far from having to husband any morsel of food consisting mainly of protein and fat, our bodies often have to deal with an excess of carbohydrate, as we tend to eat three or four times a day and may have sugary snacks between times, too! It is a very different situation for our regulatory hormones. The vast change is bound to have its effect and it does: namely, in the sometimes subtle, sometimes dramatic manifestations of what I call the 'carbohydrate effect'.

Fat in our food has its own way of being dealt with, whereas when carbohydrates are digested they reach the bloodstream as sugar. It is the hormone insulin which is called on to deal with any excess of sugar. Apart from promoting fat storage, another thing that happens when insulin is raised is that the growth hormone soon falls and vice versa. A constantly (or too frequently) raised insulin level, i.e. without adequate pauses between meals and snacks containing carbohydrate, means a constantly (or too frequently) depressed level of growth hormone which, in turn, affects the health of our immune system and has an adverse affect on the maintenance of our tissues. Many damaging consequences for our body are likely to follow from this, including weak muscles and poor connective tissue, osteoporosis, arteriosclerosis and reduced resistance to stress, infection and possibly to cancer, to name but a few.

The fat we eat makes no such demands on our insulin supply and so does not result in a depression of the growth hormone. As long as the quantity of carbohydrate is kept sufficiently low, dietary fat supplies us with the calories we need without these damaging consequences to our body tissues.

SO YOU SEE, CALORIES ARE NOT JUST CALORIES WHATEVER THEIR SOURCE!

Q: So you think it wrong to cut down fat and eat more carbohydrate?

Dr Lutz: Definitely, in my experience it is quite the wrong way round. You see, the further we get from an active outdoor life and a meat-based diet, the less we function according to our design and the more strain we put upon our regulators. Think of it like this: because of our origins, our bodies are best suited to eating food from the animal kingdom on a regular basis (with or without the addition of some plant food): hormonally speaking, a huge regular influx of carbohydrate foods constitutes an emergency situation.

Now, an emergency squad should be for occasional call-out and then go back to base when the trouble is over. To enable us to cope with an occasional high carbohydrate food, our hormones can and do pull out emergency stops, and this works all right. They can even cope with a moderate intake of carbohydrate by prioritising the need to deal with it, and then getting back to their regular working.

But a constant flood of carbohydrate coming into the system

necessitates constant emergency call-out, with little on no respite. My medical work has amply shown that even the measures our hormones undertake to accommodate this latter situation can predispose us to illness. The strain and hormonal exhaustion that tend to follow can also manifest in disease: one way or another, the system eventually breaks down and the cost to our health is high.

At bottom, we need to eat that quantity of carbohydrate which protects the blood sugar regulatory system to such an extent that the chances of exhaustion and hence the danger not only of diabetes but of other diseases associated with hormonal regulation are reduced to a minimum. This we can only do by keeping our carbohydrate intake low enough and including enough fat in our food. It is a problem Western medicine has not come to grips with yet.

Q: So, Dr Lutz, are you saying that carbohydrates are bad for us?

Dr Lutz: What I am saying is that the regular eating of more than a certain amount of carbohydrate can be, as you put it, 'bad for us'.

Q: Is this 'certain amount' the same amount for everyone?

Dr Lutz: Not necessarily – how much the body can manage without too much harm and for how long depends to some extent on our constitution, as well as on individual exercise level, medical history and any damage already done. It may also depend on our genes, as heredity seems to play a part. More work is needed on this point.

Q: Dr Lutz, may I ask how you can tell that I, personally, am eating too much carbohydrate?

Dr Lutz: Unfortunately, by the medical condition that brings you here to see me.

Q: Dr Lutz, should we all be on your diet – my whole family, kids and all?

Dr Lutz: Ideally yes, and for the best results, I feel it is particularly important to start carbohydrate restriction as soon in life as possible. It is also a lot easier and more congenial if all the family participate.

And as to fat – who would ever think of putting, say, a two-year old on something as unnatural as a low fat diet? Ridiculous!

Q: In terms of diet, is merely restricting carbohydrate enough, in itself, to maintain health?

Dr Lutz: It may be, that is if enough protein and fat are eaten, but there are necessarily other factors involved. For instance, I personally find increasing benefit from additionally restricting salt intake. When patients are well established on my diet, even when they have been previously short of, say, iron or calcium, I have seldom found the need to prescribe vitamin or mineral supplements. One must remember, however, that the diet is by no means a cure-all, especially if started later on in life.

The reason I, as a doctor, have concentrated on carbohydrate restriction is because I have witnessed over half a lifetime the fundamental contribution this one measure alone can make both to treating illness and to overall health. I would go further than this and say that curbing excessive carbohydrate intake is essential to good health. Of course, 'excessive' is a relative concept: relative to each individual's present condition, and which has reference to his or her past and as well as to the future. Nevertheless, I stand by what I say about the necessity for curbing excess.

Q: Does one have to go right down to 72g of carbohydrate daily?

Dr Lutz: One of the lovely things about this way of eating is that, almost as soon as they start cutting down, people often start to feel better in themselves. For those in the habit of overindulgence in carbohydrates, even a small reduction can be beneficial. I grant you that a successful compromise is often found at 7, 8, 9 or even 10 bread units.

Some of my patients stay well on slightly more than 72g, a few even on 100–120g, though there tends to be a breaking point above which relapse occurs. What I myself have found from years of clinical practice is that there are some medical conditions for which good and lasting results can only be obtained if carbohydrate is reduced to, and often kept for a long while, at the amount I recommend.

I have not given much attention to, shall we say, a medium level of carbohydrate as a long-term proposition, nor to the considerable variation there exists between what individuals seem to tolerate without harm. Both of these topics I must leave to others.

Q: Isn't reducing carbohydrate to 72g a day a bit extreme?

Dr Lutz: On the contrary, it is extreme to eat the huge amount of carbohydrate that many people do today. It is this excess, which I feel causes such problems with our health. The guideline of 72g daily – or thereabouts – is the amount I have found generally most suitable for therapeutic purposes.

I say 'therapeutic purposes' because, as a physician, my concern has been in treating people who in all likelihood were, as I said, already suffering from the consequences of carbohydrate overload and who often also had a hereditary predisposition to certain illnesses through their parents and grandparents. My task has been to find out how much reduction in carbohydrate intake was sufficient with individual patients to counteract the carbohydrate effect I was observing and so to avert its various adverse manifestations. With my obese hyperinsulinic teenagers, for instance, I found that 72 – 80g of carbohydrate was the maximum they could tolerate without relapse.

Q: But Dr Lutz, our society is dependent on mental achievement. I myself am a city-dweller and a brain-worker*, surely my efficiency depends on my brain getting enough carbohydrate?

Dr Lutz: Yes, in our society, the brain generally does use carbohydrate – glucose – for its fuel. This can come from dietary carbohydrate, or this sugar can be made from protein (from our food or from waste body proteins); it can even be made from fat*. Anyone living on my diet will have enough protein from which to make sugar if needed. However, the brain can run happily on ketone bodies instead of glucose. In many years of observation, I have never found evidence that the brain suffers in any way, so presumably it is able to cover its nutritional needs from the diet.

Q: How can I tell if I have cut down carbohydrates sufficiently?

Dr Lutz: You will know you are on the right lines when you stop having dental fillings and your dentist surprises you by praising the firmness of your gums! Or perhaps when you have fewer infections or your corns disappear – it all depends on your weak spots. Sometimes there are gains in health where you least expect them. Improvement can show itself, for example, in the loss of indigestion or other abdominal discomfort, or in the warming up of habitually cold hands and feet.

In minor illness, you will know when your symptoms start to abate. In serious illness, this naturally depends on what you are suffering from and it may take time: here you would be under my guidance or under the supervision of another doctor.

Always hungry

Q: Dr Lutz, why is it that I am always so hungry?

Dr Lutz: Sweet and starchy items of food are what we call 'morish' for the simple reason that the more you eat of them, the more you want to eat of them and the more you think you need. The underlying reason for this is called hyperinsulinism – the body pours out too much insulin, in effect dealing a little too energetically with the excess of sugar you have confronted it with from the carbohydrate in your food, which is now sugar in your blood. This can result in a temporary shortage of sugar in the bloodstream and consequently in a recurrence of feeling hungry, even soon after a meal.

Q: Dr Lutz, if I keep feeling hungry, shouldn't I eat something sweet?

Dr Lutz: The problem needs tackling at its roots: that is, that you have been in the habit of eating too much carbohydrate. The first step is to make sure that you have some protein and fat at each meal. If you have been having just toast and marmalade for breakfast, you will be wanting biscuits at eleven, so the thing to do is to try eating something for breakfast that 'lines your stomach', as it were, and that lasts until lunch: like bacon and egg, with only one slice of toast and marmalade and without a dish of cereal to start with.

Initially, you may still feel the need to snack between meals. If so, it is preferable to snack on something containing mostly protein and fat – say a few nuts or a piece of cold sausage. Once you stop having so many sweet or starchy things, the problem should gradually go away. Then you will no longer be 'always hungry', but only want to eat when your body genuinely needs food, which is a very peaceful experience. Of course, you might have to limit your tea and coffee and other such stimulants, too!

Q: Can one ever lose one's sweet tooth on your diet?

Dr Lutz: Some people do so, though I confess I've never lost mine. However, the occasional pastry or dessert (which is within-bounds as to the daily quota of carbohydrate) becomes all the more delightful for being a rare treat!

Q: What about this business of 60% or more of your calories having to come from carbohydrate?

Dr Lutz: Percentages are very misleading – what does such a percentage look like on the dinner plate? Of course, you have no idea. Well, your body does not recognise percentages either, only amounts!

Long term?

Q: There are so many diets to chose from, Dr Lutz. We are told that it is best to eat a low fat, high carbohydrate diet; others say vegetarian is best; others that grain is bad or that grain is good!

Dr Lutz: There are a great many factors which can mar or improve our health. I know that, in terms of diet, I have not said the last word that is to be said.

What I do say, however, is let those who put forward their particular ideas of diet spend as many years and as much effort as I have done watching the effect of their diets on real individuals over a great many years. Let them also perform a great number of clinical tests to ensure that their diets result in good liver function, in healthy levels of triglycerides, cholesterol and other blood fats, in normal blood pressure and in the reduction of chronic inflammation. Let them show actual improvements for example in enzyme reactions in hepatic diseases or in the EEG of angina pectoris patients.

In short, let them seek sufficient evidence that their diet can alleviate or cure one or the other disease and much more besides – that it can not only help restore health but also help keep people healthy, and do this in the long term.

Q: Is this diet a diet or a permanent way of eating, Dr Lutz?

Dr Lutz: There are many different diets around, some very successful in the short term and people therefore feel they 'work'. Take fasting: it can be an excellent measure for losing weight, but it is necessarily a temporary measure and going back to the old habits afterward can mean the weight piles on again. What matters is that people adopt a way of eating which satisfies the appetite and which will still be effective in maintaining their health not just for a few weeks or months but in, say, thirty or forty years time.

I call my method a 'diet' for convenience, but as regards the paucity of carbohydrate content, it certainly used to be a permanent way of eating in the distant past! In this part of the world, it is only recently – in the last few thousand and, in some countries, few hundred years – that carbohydrate foods have become the main staple.

As to the long-term nature of the diet, you will find the answer in your own improved health, whilst you stay on this level of carbohydrate. You might also have this same answer reinforced when, sad to say, you have a relapse into your old illness as a result of a sudden carbohydrate binge or just by regularly upping the level too much.

Q: Is it safe to eat so little carbohydrate for so long?

Dr Lutz: In general, my diet is very safe as a long-term way of eating and very protective of your health. You see, you will probably be eating a very modest amount of food altogether, so there will be no danger of over-eating. If you satisfy your appetite on the permitted foods, you will also be getting enough of the materials you need to build and maintain your body in good health, without the sort of troubles that are induced by overeating in general and of starchy and sugary foods in particular.

Q: Does this mean that we should eat meat every day?

Dr Lutz: I am not saying that one has to eat meat every day, but nor am I saying that it is harmful to do so. Meat is a valuable source of nutrients and it has been an integral part of our way of eating for a very long time. When the fat is included, meat is a complete food: indeed, one can be healthy just on fresh fat meat, but there is no need for such an extreme. I am not dogmatic about the menu as long as carbohydrate is kept at a suitably low level. Many people wish to eat a little meat, fish or dairy food at each meal and that is fine.

Entertaining and eating out

Q: Would you recommend minimalism, Dr Lutz?

Dr Lutz: I think it an excellent idea when applied to carbohydrates! In fact, it is a very good way for people on my diet to entertain in gourmet style – a wealth of tiny tempting dishes, most of them savoury together with exquisite tiny deserts, more works of art than fillers. Yes, you would have happy guests and probably no one would suspect a 'diet' or notice any absence of carbohydrate.

Q: How shall I cope with eating out, Dr Lutz?

Dr Lutz: In a restaurant, it is usually possible to avoid the starchiest dishes, to have the antipasto rather than the pasta for example, or to eat a good serving of roast meat with spinach and mushrooms à la crème but to take only one potato.

Q: Most of my friends are on high carbohydrate, low fat diets, so what do I do when I visit them?

Dr Lutz: When you are at home, you can make your own choices. If, at a friend's house, there is no choice but spaghetti on toast, followed by chocolate biscuits – and it does happen – you accept a very modest portion and cut down on carbohydrates for the rest of the day. Of course, it may be possible to take the friend into your confidence and explain simply that you are 'under doctor's orders'. Other food may then be forthcoming, next time at least!

Sugar

Q: Should one avoid all sugar?

Dr Lutz: Certainly, one ought to limit the amount. Sugar that comes in a packet is a very concentrated carbohydrate and there is quite a lot of it hidden in commercially prepared foods. I find that some of my patients can tolerate it in small amounts; some cannot even have any at all without a return of their symptoms. You see, sugar can be quite brutal, especially in its effects on the upper part of the digestive tract: cutting it out entirely can sometimes lead to a lessening or cessation of symptoms in just a few days. I am thinking here of conditions such as heartburn.

And bread?

Q: Surely our ancestors would have nibbled wild grass seeds as they walked though the countryside, like the disciples of Jesus?

Dr Lutz: Very probably – if they were hungry enough, that is! But it takes an enormous amount of nibbling of grass seeds to ingest any appreciable amount of carbohydrate. Also, it seems it is only since the last Ice Age that genetic mutation has led to strains of wheat suitable for cultivation by man. It is highly probable that cereals only began to be eaten in any quantity when they could be sown, reaped and stored, that is during the last few thousand years.

Q: What about bread, Dr Lutz, is that better than sweet foods?

Dr Lutz: Well, what I have just said about sweet foods also applies to bread. My patients tell me it is perhaps the most 'morish' of foods: one occasional thin slice becomes two regular ones, then three, then four and before they know it they have doubled their daily bread units and are wondering why they no longer feel so well. Many of my patients find it easier to do without bread entirely.

Q: If I do eat bread, should I prefer wholemeal bread, Dr Lutz?

Dr Lutz: Not necessarily. In principle, it is better and more natural than white bread, but it really depends on how happy your gut is after eating it. For anyone suffering from disorders of the intestines, I find wholemeal bread is one of the least tolerated foods. Others may eat a very moderate amount of it, if they like.

The question of wholefood

Q: Dr Lutz, you are not known particularly as a 'wholefooder' or one belonging to the organic lobby. Would it be true to say you are against the idea of wholefood.

Dr Lutz: On the contrary, I have always felt it to be a truism that food does not improve in quality by being refined or otherwise being denatured. As long ago as 1970, I remember writing that I took all that for granted. Yes, of course we should eat food that is as whole and as natural as possible – and what more whole and more natural than fresh fat meat!

Q: Dr Lutz, are you sure that it is the quantity of carbohydrate eaten that makes the difference? Would not eating whole food produce equal results?

Dr Lutz: It is difficult to dissociate the effect of refinement from the problems of increase in carbohydrate per se, as they go hand in hand. But I am quite sure that it is not just wholeness that matters, especially when it is a question of repairing damage caused by past excess.

The important thing is the composition of the diet: apart from things like water, minerals, vitamins and trace elements, to my mind, A DIET SUITED TO REGAIN OR MAINTAIN HEALTH REQUIRES FIRSTLY ENOUGH PROTEIN AND FAT, SECONDLY (AND SPECIFICALLY) NOT TOO MUCH CARBOHYDRATE OF ANY SORT. This is the message that comes though loud and clear from my entire medical work in this field.

222

Note: **ENOUGH DOES NOT IMPLY THAT PROTEIN AND FAT NECESSARILY HAVE TO BE CONSUMED IN LARGE AMOUNTS.** Individual requirements as to quantity vary widely according to age, exercise level etc.

Q: Dr Lutz, just to clarify this point still further, are you saying that carbohydrates can still be harmful, even if they are whole, organically grown and even raw?

Dr Lutz: Precisely. Mind you, eating so-called wholefood may mean you eat less carbohydrate in total, but not necessarily so.

So, yes, if they are eaten in excess, and I mean excess for that particular individual, carbohydrates in any form can be harmful. I found this with my chicken experiments: there was nothing 'unwhole' about the diet of the chickens that were eating high carbohydrate feed – they were even eating their wheat as whole grains – but this did not prevent arteriosclerosis developing nor did it prevent them getting obese. It was the hens that had less carbohydrate altogether that fared so much better in these respects.

I am fairly sure that the picture is the same with humans. I know, for example, that merely cutting out sugar did not improve the condition of my Crohn's patients, only reducing carbohydrate from every source.

Q: Dr Lutz, forgive me for persisting, but you say that wholemeal bread is a problem and that food should be as whole as possible. Is that not a contradiction?

Dr Lutz: I think perhaps you misunderstand what I am saying. Being close to nature and her laws is what my dietary therapy is all about. Being a very recent food in the human diet, grain is not, as often supposed, our original staple. So when I talk of good fresh food, I am not necessarily referring to the bread one can very well do without – far from it! You see, when nature's laws have been long unheeded and the body is struggling to make the best of things, then special measures may be needed to redress existing damage.

If you cut a finger, you guard it against further harm at least until it has a chance to heal and possibly longer. Well, it is the same when I advise my bowel patients to avoid fibre-rich wholemeal bread or other foods that may irritate an organ that is already irritated. Only after much improvement should one expose it to potential irritants and then cautiously. And there are some people whom bread, and especially wholemeal bread, just does not suit.

Q: Dr Lutz, so you allow refined food in your diet?

Dr Lutz: Shall we say rather that I encourage my patients to respect the antiquity of human eating habits: I advise them, for instance, to eat good proteins and good natural fats, especially of animal origin. I discourage the use of margarines and any other over-processed fats, including refined cooking oils.

On a limit of 72g or so of carbohydrate, I do not find it important to be strict on the issue of refinement. I try to be firm in what I think really matters and to allow enough individual choice in anything that matters less. The diet is easier that way – and kinder, too!

Fruit and vegetables

Q: Dr Lutz, what about fruit and vegetables?

Dr Lutz: They may be included in reasonable quantities. However, I urge moderation with starchy vegetables and especially with fruit. In general, fruit and vegetables are a useful supplement to the basic diet, but it is important to realise that you can have too much even of a supposed 'good' thing.

Q: On your diet, may I still have the recommended five pieces of fruit and vegetable a day?

Dr Lutz: Fruit can contain a surprising amount of carbohydrate. But, if it suits you, it is fine to do so – that is, as long as it is possible to eat five pieces of fruit and still keep within the daily carbohydrate ration. Within this limit, the choice is yours.

Modern dilemma

Q: What would you say is the basis of your dietary approach in treating illness?

Dr Lutz: When patients cut down their carbohydrate intake as instructed, it is as though their bodies move into a different and healthier gear in which healing somehow becomes more possible. Basically, what I try to do is to cut down carbohydrate sufficiently to elicit this change, with its calming, normalising and restorative effect on the body.

Q: What do you see as normal, Dr Lutz?

Dr Lutz: Do we really know? I am a doctor who, albeit a pioneer and a bit of a rebel, has worked within the framework of Western medicine all his life: so by 'normal', I refer for instance to the accepted laboratory values of this culture. Of course, carbohydrate restriction as a sole measure does not necessarily achieve what we want it to: there being always many factors involved that affect the outcome. Some abnormalities, for example, may be symptoms of serious underlying disease.

However, though things are not always straightforward, I have been able to demonstrate the tendency of my diet to bring body functions back into line, as I have shown in regard to problems with blood sugar, blood pressure, triglycerides, cholesterol, uric acid, sex hormone levels, stomach acid and more. This tendency to normalise is one of the striking things about the diet and why it is such a useful tool for the practising physician. I have found that there is a whole range of medical conditions, including some liver and heart problems, which respond well to low carbohydrate nutrition.

Q: Dr Lutz, why do you think so many different conditions respond to low carbohydrate nutrition?

Dr Lutz: I feel that this way of eating provides all the necessary materials for maintaining and repairing our bodies, as well as providing the necessary fuel.

You see, for any particular engine, if you use the wrong fuel, there will be trouble. Use the right one and, unless too much damage is already done, the engine then functions more efficiently and gives a lot less trouble – it also lasts longer! At its simplest, I think one of the reasons that my diet is such an effective therapy in so many widely different diseases is its capacity to restore more efficient functioning by giving it the right fuel, as it were.

Naturally, it is not that simple as the body is a self-repairing 'engine', which runs on a mixture of fuels. However, the internal fuel mix that the body derives from a low carbohydrate diet is more appropriate to the needs of the body than that derived from a diet too high in carbohydrate. There is a lot more research needed to clarify all the connections but, briefly, on the more suitable fuel mix that my diet provides, it seems that the body struggles less to make-do, stress is reduced and, overall, things tend to work better.

Healing then not only becomes more possible but a great many patients are enabled to lead a better life. I have written at length about my medical work in my other books.

Q: What, then, is your opinion of the standard nutritional advice?

Dr Lutz: That, sadly, the standard advice is not only flawed but is actually creating more of the very conditions the advice is trying to prevent. The mistake of seeing carbohydrates as the basis (and largest component) of a health-giving diet, and the resultant overconsumption of carbohydrates, has led to widespread malnutrition and, tragically, to the mushrooming of Type-II obesity, diabetes, cancer and many other serious health problems*.

Q: Dr Lutz, in your opinion, is there a way out of the maze in which you say current nutritional thinking has found itself?

Dr Lutz: Well, if you need to find your way out of a maze, the thing to do is to keep calm, think straight – and it helps if you are tall enough to see over the hedges! It is the same with diet: we need to take a long view, that is to get away from the clutter of detail and develop a perspective on diet based on our evolutionary history and one which is backed by sound biology. We shall think straighter if we remember four points:

1. that, as we evolved, our original diet consisted, perhaps not exclusively, but for the large part of protein and fat of animal origin and this gives a clue to the internal requirements of our bodily constitution
2. that a moderate amount of carbohydrate can still be compatible with these requirements – the body can use some of it as sugar and easily convert the rest into fat, the fuel it needs and by and large prefers
3. that all warm-blooded animals have a limit to the amount of carbohydrate they can eat without upsetting their health – the point at which insulin has to prioritise too often the use of sugar as a fuel, which requires disadvantageous adjustments from our whole hormonal system
4. that the average daily intake of carbohydrates in the Western world already exceeds this limit and that the intake of some individuals exceeds it by far.

In my various books, I discuss in detail the many and sometimes subtle detrimental changes that can happen to our body processes, our hormones and to our health when this limit is regularly exceeded. So, yes, I do think there is a way out and, in my own mind, I am sure that carbohydrate restriction points the way.

Q: So how do you feel about Robert Atkins, Dr Lutz?

Dr Lutz: I think it is wonderful to see such a rush of enthusiasm for low carbohydrate nutrition and to read of so many people feeling the better for it.

Q: Dr Lutz, what do you think of the so-called 'Atkins' diet'?

Dr Lutz: Not so wonderful! You see, it can be dangerous to cut out all or even most carbohydrate suddenly. The young and fit may perhaps do so with impunity, but people who are older or who are unwell can make themselves ill or even court disaster by doing so.

A blanket recommendation for combating obesity this way, whatever the age and condition of the patient is, in my view, downright irresponsible. The body needs time to adjust to such a drastic change of diet. My more gentle approach is very different to that of my late colleague.

Q: There seem many types of diet that have been shown to maintain good health, including vegetarian and wholefood organic, which is natural and unadulterated.

Dr Lutz: The importance of good quality foodstuff is not under dispute. What we must realise is that we can eat an amazing variety of foods and still be healthy. This is mainly because of the wonderful means our body has of converting the ingredients in food into the materials it needs for its internal functioning. So it is not just a question of, say, should we eat meat or not, should we eat grain or not, should we avoid all cow produce or not (though there may be valid subsidiary reasons for doing or not doing any of these things). It is rather a question of discovering (and then acknowledging) the parameters within which the body can deal unharmed with any particular composition of diet.

In terms of nutrition, I might go further and suggest that, individual idiosyncrasies apart, health depends to a large extent on the composition of the food we regularly eat coming within these parameters. Surely this is the common ground which unites all diets that support excellent physique: that they have enough protein and fat to meet bodily needs, a variable amount of carbohydrate, but not so much as to hinder the proper utilisation of the protein and fat? Western medicine already acknowledges that one can have too little protein for health, it is beginning to recognise the problems of having too much sugar and refined carbohydrate (though not yet of total carbohydrate), however it is currently still very confused about the problems of eating too little fat, especially saturated fat!

The way forward

Q: Dr Lutz, many of us have spent years eating a lot of carbohydrate foods and are already showing some of the signs of the damage you mention. As a last question, may I ask you to put – in a nutshell – what we can do about it?

Dr Lutz: Redressing years of damage is not necessarily straightforward, nor is it always possible, and therefore any attempt to do so needs to be backed by thorough understanding. I must emphasise that my method is no five-day wonder: the diet takes time to have effect and is intended for regular long-term use, so that the body is given a chance to work properly. I have tried to indicate the necessary cautions, speed of change, expected results and so on in this book, and explained why anyone seriously ill needs to be under the guidance of a physician.

To prevent trouble occurring in the first place, my nutritional regime is obviously best used from birth and preferably beforehand, but we are talking of damage already done by prolonged carbohydrate excess. In a nutshell, what we can do about it is to restrict total carbohydrates (i.e. all the sugars and starches eaten in any one day) sufficiently to elicit healing. In practice, I advocate eating enough protein and fat to give the body what it needs for efficient functioning and gradually reducing the daily carbohydrate intake to a level that does not unduly disturb the balance of our endocrine hormones – and this is crucial. It is as simple and, since I am referring to the body's internal requirements, as complex as that.

The carbohydrate effect

To date, my journey of discovery has taken forty-five years. Though I did not have the facilities to do formal clinical trials, I have been in the privileged position of gaining extensive clinical experience and of being able to collect data first hand, as it were, recording lab test results and other clinical findings over substantial periods of time, sometimes over many years. This painstaking observation over half a lifetime led me to the realization of the profound influence that the level of carbohydrate in our diet has on our health, for better or for worse.

I have become ever more convinced of the extensive and insidiously corrupting influence that an overload of carbohydrate has on our health: that is, of the 'carbohydrate effect'. Naturally, I could not, in all conscience, test this effect by recommending that a group of people eat large quantities of carbohydrate and then document the results, nor could I do the same with my patients to see if their conditions were aggravated. This, to me, would be an experiment that was totally unethical. As a clinician, I could only document this effect by implication and inference: namely, by restricting carbohydrate and showing the reversal or amelioration of conditions which, directly or indirectly, I thought to be induced by excess carbohydrate in the first place.

Wittingly or not*, this experiment has nevertheless been carried out on a large scale in the Western world: namely, carbohydrate has been promoted at the expense of fat. Ostensibly, the object of this has been to combat obesity, diabetes, heart disease and cancer through the reduction of animal fat and red meat; its tactic has been that of scaremongering, especially about animal fats, based on the misinterpretation of studies and supported by a food industry that quickly adapted to the new way. Far from achieving its object, the result is all too familiar: that is, with the exception of a small drop in fatalities from heart infarcts, there has been a mushrooming of these very same diseases!

Personally, I have done what I can to show the way forward in the furtherance of health through carbohydrate restriction. It is one of the challenges of future medical science to further the understanding both of individual and general requirements in this respect.

I therefore end by urging my medical colleagues everywhere to observe and to study, to collect and to sift relevant data, to analyse, to understand and then to

COLLECTIVELY CONFRONT THE CARBOHYDRATE EFFECT.

NOTES

CHAPTER 1

Page 21 *D-I-Y instructions* Dr Lutz was a caring physician with a direct interest in those on his diet. He was aware that any change can be stressful and that people trying the diet for the first time might need help and guidance. Dr Lutz was aware, too, that people do try diets from books (see letter and comments on p 175), that they frequently ignore warnings for example about the speed of implementation and the level of carbohydrate to aim at, or as to the necessity of including enough fat. All he could do for posterity was, therefore, to record as clearly as possible his own experiences with the diet and some of what he learnt during the 50 years he was advising and guiding patients.

Page 22 *Haag am Hausruck*, a village of about 2,000 inhabitants in the district of Grieskirchen, a largely forested area in Upper Austria, about 500 metres above sea level. Hausruck is a range of mountains in the foothills of the Alps.

Page 23 *papers on the subject A* full list of scientific papers can be found in the section 'Further Publications by Dr med. habil. Wolfgang Lutz'.

Page 26 *Habilitation* is a great honour. In Germany, it is the highest academic qualification an individual can receive on their own merit; it ranks above a Ph.D. and qualifies the recipient to teach at a university.

Page 27 *internal medicine* In some countries, internal medicine is known as 'general medicine'. It is a speciality in its own right, often dealing with adult disorders of diagnostic doubt or where there are multiple conditions present, which therefore may be complex and not fit existing categories.

Page 27 *Ried im Innkreis*, a town of about 11,000, administrative centre for the province of Innviertel.

Page 31 *adrenal insufficiency* Dr Lutz thought this fitted with Weissbecker's concept of secondary adrenal insufficiency, which he does not define.

Page 32 *Herbert Kühn* was professor of prehistory at the University of Mainz. His book *Das Erwachen der Menschheit* (the awakening of humanity) was issued in translation in 1955 by Random House, New York, entitled *On the Track of Prehistoric Man.* In his tours through the caves, Kühn also mentions paintings or engravings of small creatures such as wolves, hares, birds and fish, suggesting these were also part of the Ice-Age diet. The paintings, he says, were done with oil paints i.e. ground mineral pigments such as ochre mixed with animal fat.

Page 33 *address* On 4 June 1957, Dr Thorpe gave the chairman's address to the section on general practice at 106 annual meeting of A M A, N Y. It also included the following:

> If the carbohydrate intake is held well within the capacity of the tissues to oxidise the pyruvic acid formed from it, then all the carbohydrate ingested will be completely changed to carbon dioxide and water. Restriction of carbohydrate removes the stimulus to insulin production, so that the future activity of insulin will be held to a minimum. The anterior pituitary fat-mobilising principle will then predominate over the fat-storing forces. Fat will be mobilised from the adipose deposits of the body, oxidised to ketones in the liver, and circulated to the tissues in this easily combustible form. By whatever dietary method reduction of excess weight is accomplished, this normal mechanism of ketogenesis must be brought into play, for it has long been known that, while carbohydrate can be readily converted into fat in the body, fat cannot be converted into carbohydrate in any significant amount.
>
> Thorpe (1957)

Page 36 *harsh environment* Put simply, the surface of Europe at that time was either covered in ice, tundra or coniferous forest. Talking of the ice sheets some 18,000 years ago:

> [One] ice sheet radiated out from . . . Scandinavia, reaching as far as the site of Moscow to the southeast, blanketing eastern Denmark and the northern sections of Germany and Poland, then merging in the North Sea with a smaller ice sheet that flowed from the Scottish highlands and the mountains of northern England, Wales and Ireland. Switzerland and neighbouring parts of Austria, Germany, France and Italy were buried under a mass of Alpine ice that stretched from the Rhone above Lyon to Graz

in Austria. The Pyrenees were an ice-armoured barrier between France and Spain . . .

Plant life was altered considerably by the combined assault of cold and increased aridity . . . Around the margins of the ice sheets was a zone of treeless tundra, clothed with arctic mosses, sedges, lichens and heathers. Beneath the thin skin of vegetation, which was watered by summer melting . . . the land was frozen. In some places, the freezing was permanent and this permafrost penetrated to depths of as much as 1,000 feet . . .

At the height of the last Ice Age, the European tundra belt covered southern Britain, northern France, Germany and Poland. To the east, it merged into patchy forest; to the south, it passed into a belt of cold, arid steppe that stretched from the Atlantic coast of Brittany to eastern Siberia. Small strands of birch, poplar and oak managed to survive in sheltered parts of south-central France but true forests were pushed south of the Alps and Pyrenees. Even at these lower latitudes, evergreen conifers were the dominant trees; deciduous woodlands were found no farther north than the islands of the western Mediterranean, the southern part of Greece, and the shores of the Black Sea (then a freshwater lake) and the Caspian Sea.

Chorlton (1983) page 24 + 30

Page 36 *health, strength and stature* There is considerable evidence of the robust health of our Ice-Age forbears and Dr Lutz was an avid reader of articles in this field. However, techniques in genetic research and for analysing old bones in relation to food eaten is growing ever more sophisticated. Therefore, rather than trying to summarise old findings, perhaps we ought to await the evidence these new techniques will disclose?

Page 38 *hybrid wheat* Bronowski tells that, though in the Old World some wild grasses had previously been reaped around Jericho:

Before 8,000 BC wheat was not the luxuriant plant it is today; it was merely one of many wild grasses that spread throughout the Middle East. By some genetic accident, the wild wheat crossed with a natural goat grass and formed a fertile hybrid [Emmer]. That accident must have happened many times in the springing vegetation that came up after the last Ice Age . . . The hybrid was able to spread naturally, because its seeds are attached to the husk in such a way that scatter in the wind.

. . . now the story of the rich plant life that followed the Ice Ages becomes more surprising. There was a second genetic accident . . . Emmer crossed with another natural goat grass and produced a still larger hybrid . . . which is bread wheat. That was improbable enough in itself, and we know now that bread wheat would not have been fertile but for a specific genetic mutation on one chromosome.

Yet there is something even stranger. Now we have a beautiful ear of wheat, but one which will never spread in the wind because the ear is too tight to break up . . . Suddenly man and the plant have come together . . . For the bread wheat can only multiply with help; man must harvest the ears and scatter their seeds; and the life of each, man and the plant, depends on the other.

Bronowski (1979) p 68

Page 39 *toleration of plant food* The note for Page 36 also applies to the state of health found during the transition from hunter/gathering to agriculture.

First published in 1939, *Nutrition and Physical Degeneration* (Price, 1998) gives a fascinating account of the way Neolithic foods formed part of the diets of various peoples both with and without harm to their health. It is only a pity that the actual amount of carbohydrate in such diets, though measured at the time, is not given. This lack of information highlights the problems of refinement but obscures the question of quantity, which Dr Lutz held to be also of the utmost importance. The same is true of *The Saccharine Diseases* (Cleave, 1974), which emphasises sugar as the main cause of modern disease, not the fact that, like the refining of flour, the inclusion of sugar in the diet tends to put up total carbohydrate intake.

Dr Lutz showed with his hens that a high carbohydrate diet, even when whole and unrefined could cause degenerative problems. Sir Robert McCarrison found that his Sikhs, whose staple was freshly ground whole wheat, stayed fit healthy only as long as their diet contained enough protein and fat (in this case whole milk and milk products). In *Nutrition and Health* (McCarrison, 1982) the superb physique of the Pathans of North India, who ate meat in considerable quantity, is also mentioned, but as this diet came only second in his rat feeding trials, regrettably we learn no more about their diet or their health.

CHAPTER 2

Page 41 *William Banting* The account of his spectacular conquering of obesity using a fat, protein and alcohol-containing, calorific diet, unrestricted except as to carbohydrate was written up in Banting's anonymous and now celebrated 'Letter on Corpulence' in 1864. Mackarness's book *Eat Fat and Grow Slim*, which gives a good summary of the whole saga, was in fact subtitled *'or Banting up to date'*.

Page 51 *my publications* List of publications by W J Lutz is divided between those in the References and those listed under Further Publications.

CHAPTER 3

Page 53 *von Noorden* Carl Harko von Noorden (1858 –1944) was professor of internal medicine at the University of Vienna from 1906.

Page 62 *insatiable desire for food* Dr Lutz showed how when hyperinsulinism was present the blood sugar tended to fall too low: i.e. below the normal bounds and said this explained the frequent cravings for sweet or starchy foods exhibited by these children before going on the diet. See Q & A: p 216-7.

Page 64 *unnecessary to restrict calories* In relation to obesity, this sentiment was echoed at this time by Mackarness:

> *It is excess carbohydrates and not calories only that make a fat man fat.* The tiresome business of totting up daily calories, on which most modern reducing diets are based, is a waste of time for an obese person. Because, as Professor Kekwick and Dr Pawan showed, a fat man may maintain his weight on a low calorie diet, if it is taken mainly as carbohydrate, but he will lose weight on a much higher calorie diet *provided he eats it mainly in the form of fat and protein.*
>
> Mackarness (1958)

Page 68 *sex hormones* In the other books by Dr Lutz, there is some confusion over the effect of carbohydrates on sex hormones. On the one hand, his own research had shown that raised oestrogen levels reduced with carbohydrate reduction. On the other, Dr Lutz found that the more overweight his youngsters were, the fewer sex hormones they produced in the run up to puberty, but this does not imply that carbohydrates diminish sex hormone production per se, as has been suggested in both *Leben ohne Brot* and *Life without Bread*. It may merely mean that the obesity of these children somehow inhibited the production of a normal quantity of sex hormones in the first place and so delayed sexual maturation. Indeed, that excessive carbohydrate consumption encourages early puberty and increases fertility is well known: Dr Lutz himself mentions this in connection with the historical transition to cereal cultivation and so to a more carbohydrate-rich diet; it was also demonstrated in his chicken experiments.

Thus there is no intrinsic contradiction in his actual findings. In relation to insulin, Dr Lutz described the process whereby a diet leading to the excessive stimulation of hormones can lead to overproduction (in this case hyperinsulinism), how this overproduction can become fixed, leading to insulin resistance (early stage diabetes) and also how this can be followed by decreased production when a stage of exhaustion is reached (late stage diabetes). Perhaps the same process of overstimulation and eventual exhaustion is at work with sex hormones, namely with carbohydrates initially promoting increased fertility but eventually leading to infertility? That this may operate both within the lifetime of an individual and over generations is also a possibility. Much more work is needed on this whole area.

Page 69 *gradually faded* The fading of striae was much faster in young people. Very marked striae present in adults with greatly increased cortisol metabolite excretion could take a long time to fade. Dr Lutz talks of one patient with morbus Cushing whom he put on a low carbohydrate diet and whose striae were much less pronounced after nine years, though still visible; however, the patient felt much better in himself much sooner than that. See colour photo on p 348 of *Dismantling a Myth.*

Page 70 *body fats* Fat is an essential part of our body structure and integral to our health and well-being. Richard Mackarness was later to put the issue very succinctly:

> The primitive hunter in pursuit of food uses exactly the same nerve signals as the NASA scientist programming computers which guide a landing on the moon. The difference is only in complexity. In both cases, the work is done by the same basic materials, chiefly animal fats. No nervous system has ever been built of starch or sugar and to base a diet on carbohydrates, as millions do today, is to invite the problems of inadequately constructed and malfunctioning brain and nerves.
>
> Mackarness (1976) p 41

Page 74 *atherosclerosis* This term refers to a form of arteriosclerosis in which there is fatty degeneration of the middle coat of the arterial wall (Blacks Medical Dictionary, 1971). In this text, atherosclerosis and arteriosclerosis are used interchangeably.

CHAPTER 4

Page 82 *A modern 'Paleolithic' diet* This is not to be confused with the recent array of Paleo diets, which are not representative of the thinking of Dr Lutz.

Page 86 *angiopathy* Dr Lutz defines angiopathy as the overgrowth of tissue e.g. in the inner layers of the blood vessels with proliferation and thickening of the basal membrane, with destruction of the smallest vessels especially in the nerves, kidney and retina. He suggests this might have its origin in excessive level of growth hormone level when insulin production became insufficient.

Page 93 *Mislimov* This story is quoted in Dismantling a Myth but no source is given. It is interesting to note that, in Wikipaedia, the myth has been recently amended: namely that Shirali Mislimov really lived not on boiled chicken but rather on fruit and vegetables, all of which he grew himself, together with wholemeal bread, chicken broth, low-fat cheese (sic) and yoghurt. Given he was a former shepherd and subsequently a member of a collective farm in the mountains in a remote village 2,000 metres above sea level with no approach road, one wonders at the veracity of this revision.

Note: an Indian man, dubbed the world's oldest father, aged 90 (with photo of him and baby) attributes his continued virility to daily walks and lots of meat: 'I eat all kinds of meat – rabbits, lamb, chicken and wild animals.' (The Scotsman, 22.8.2007)

CHAPTER 5

Page 108 *amount of fat* One the sayings of Dr Lutz was 'there is no healing of the gut without fat', and this included the tendency to constipation. Adding extra fat as a remedy for constipation is mentioned by Donaldson.

Page 112 *aggravation of symptoms* The job of the immune system, says Dr Lutz, is not just to combat infection, but to clear up the damaged tissue that the infection has caused; the breaking down and removing of damaged tissue can in itself aggravate the situation and lead to chronic inflammation.

Page 113 *gold* Gold has long been used in the treatment of tuberculosis and chronic rheumatic diseases. Toxic in large doses, it is still sometimes given in minute doses in the treatment of rheumatoid arthritis. When he felt it appropriate, Dr Lutz used it in the treatment of some auto-immune diseases during the transition phases to a low carbohydrate diet in order to subdue excessive reaction by the immune system.

Page 118 *fibre* Further light is shone on the somewhat problematic role of fibre by Heaton (1973) who suggests that fibre blocks nutrient intake in three ways: by displacing available nutrients; by slowing intake and promoting satiety by the need for chewing; by reducing the absorptive efficiency of the small intestine. Thus fibre is seen by Heaton as beneficial for obese overeaters of refined carbohydrate but, of course, may not be so for modest eaters on a 'Lutz diet'.

Page 125 D Y Each letter quoted was shared with me by Dr Lutz. No address was given on this particular letter; Dr Lutz was well acquainted with the writer. 1995 could be an error.

CHAPTER 6

Page 134 *butter yellow* Methyl yellow, known as butter yellow, is a chemical that was used to colour butter before it was suspected of being a carcinogen.

Page 135 *three component theory* From this, Dr Lutz derived – and adopted as his own – his somewhat problematic 'two component theory' to illustrate and explain the hormonal imbalances resulting from carbohydrate excess. Dr Lutz ignored the intricate interplay both at cellular level and between the various organs between the three components, seeing just the balance between the catabolic and anabolic as important. Of this oversimplified rendering of his theory, Schole always remained highly critical.

Page 136 *adaptation to stress* Hans Selye was professor of physiology at Montreal University. It was suggested in our joint book that the effect of carbohydrate as a 'noxious agent' or a 'stress' could be seen in the light of the three phases of Hans Selye's adaptation syndrome: alarm, adaptation with increased resistance and finally exhaustion.

Dr Lutz recognised the addictive quality of carbohydrate, which fitted in with phase two of the body's response to threats to its stability. Selye is explained well in the book *Not All in the Mind* by Richard Mackarness, who says about phase three:

> Patients do not generally consult their doctors until they are entering the stage of exhaustion in their struggle to adapt to an environmental stress. Lacking the means of turning back the clock in the patient's illness, the doctor is left to speculate on causes and to treat symptoms empirically as they arise.
>
> Mackarness (1976)

This late stage at which patients came to see Dr Lutz might explain why carbohydrate had to be so severely restricted and why Wolfgang Lutz gave no time to studying any middle way.

Page 142 *excess fluid* In the case of the nurse with heart failure, there is some variation in the different accounts, e.g. as to whether diuretics or drugs other than gold were or were not administered. The fact of her early death was told me as one of Dr Lutz's 'confessions' when I asked what he regretted during his long career. Here, it was not the case that many months were taken in going over to a low carbohydrate regime because, as he said, her condition was life threatening and treatment was urgent.

Page 146 *variation of intake* In Kasper, Lutz & Wild, the following figures are given: the average intake for protein was 102.6g (plus or minus 39.7g), the actual range being from 48.3g (plus or minus 8.6g) to 178.3g (plus or minus 29.3g); for fat the average intake was 156.1 (plus or minus 64.0g), the range being from 77.5g (plus or minus 26.5g) to 279.6g (plus or minus 68g); for carbohydrate the average daily intake was 74.6 (plus or minus 34.2), the range being from 44.3 (plus or minus 13.1g) to 139.2 (plus or minus 31.5).

The ranges were considerable, also as regards calories with the 22-year-old man taking more than double the calories taken by the 9-year-old girl.

Page 147 *hardback edition* The book *Dismantling a Myth,* issued by Charles Thomas, is available through the British Library lending division.

Page 148 *big American field studies* For example, in Framingham, after extensive research, the Diet Study Group reported:

> There is no indication of a relationship between dietary cholesterol and serum cholesterol. . . If the intake of animal fat is held constant there is still no relation of cholesterol intake to serum cholesterol.
>
> Gordon T (1971) 24–8

Despite this finding, the Study Group concludes that this does not mean in might be different, say, in Japan but:

> Still less does it mean that serum cholesterol levels cannot be changed by changes in dietary intake.
>
> Gordon T (1971) 24–14

This undoubtedly true statement was partly what led both to the ignoring and subsequent misquoting of some of the actual findings of Framingham, such as the important one quoted above. A good resumé of the complexities of these erroneous interpretations is given by Walter Yellowlees (1993).

Mann as ex-director of Framingham was so disillusioned by the misrepresentation of the study results that, with others, he founded the Veritas Society, explicitly to 'focus our objections and call for a return to scientific and informational honesty'. Mann edited Coronary Heart Disease (1993) for the Veritas Society. Since Mann's death in 2013, there is a society of the same name focussed on magic.

For further information on the fat theory and cholesterol, please see T H I N C S: the website of The International Network of Cholesterol Skeptics:

Page 150 two *million years* Here 'mankind' in Glatzel's phrase refers to the genus of Homo over the whole Paleolithic period or Stone Age i.e. Homo erectus, Homo Neanderthalis as well as the subsequent modern species: Homo sapiens of the Upper Paleolithic.

Page 151 *in warm climates* In his chapter 'Living off the Fat of the Land' in *Not by Bread alone* p 132, Stefansson gives examples of how necessary fat was to people in the tropics.

CHAPTER 7

Page 154 *beliefs* Stefansson himself reports:

> At Red River on July 20, 1906, I saw my first Eskimos. They were not at all as my book learning about the north had led me to believe they would be. I had expected them to be short and fat. When I saw them standing among white men on the river bank I was surprised to find them all about the same height. Still under the spell of my book of knowledge, I thought it strange that there should be such short white men in the north. When I went to the shore, I found, of course, that the men, white and Eskimo alike were as tall as or taller than I, and I am just under six feet. One thing I noticed about the Eskimo . . . was their graceful, swinging walk . . .
>
> Stefansson (1964) p 69

Page 155 *Alexander Berglas,* says that, after thirty years in the field, he concluded that one should look for the cause of cancer in our environment and mode of life. In his Epilogue, he says:

> I believe that, like every process in nature, cancer is, in the beginning, a natural functional process, a healing process, whose task is to defend the organism by all available means against a chronic attack. If this attempted healing gives rise to a malignant tumor, it is not a meaningless accident but merely an exaggeration of the process it was trying to help . . .

> Cancer, just as all other natural phenomena, obeys the rules of
> nature.
>
> Berglas (1957) p 125

Note: it was the Inuit habit of spending their indoor evenings and nights either completely naked or naked from the waist upwards which, during his early travels, enabled Stefansson to surmise the absence of breast cancer.

Later Stefansson was to write a most interesting book *Cancer: Disease of Civilisation* (1960), which was digitalised by the University of Mitchigan in 2008. There is now a copy in the British Library. It was his last book, appearing shortly before his death; in it, Stefansson had collected documentary evidence to show that the Eskimos, prior to their contact with American civilization, did not suffer from cancer. At the northern mission stations, which had been erected near the whaling stations by white people, the missionaries kept exact records of the cause of death among the natives. Stefansson was able to contact many of these ministers or their widows and, from the material he collected, it did indeed appear that there was no cancer amongst the 'natural' i.e. meat and fish-eating Eskimo.

Page 161 *calories from carbohydrate* This accords with the 2% of calories from carbohydrate found in the pre-modern Inuit diet by Draper (1978). It comes from *Discovery* p 289.

Page 162 *fat starvation* An excellent account of the need for fat in an all animal food diet and the consequences of a lack of fat is given in Stefansson (1946), especially chapter six 'Living off the Fat of the Land' pp 112–142. Stefansson explains, for example, that the Inuit can live off seal meat all year because there is enough fat on a seal to provide a balanced diet, and also enough fat for heating, lighting and cooking, whereas caribou seldom has enough fat for all these purposes, hence the need to visit the coastal areas to go seal hunting in the winter. The chapter includes examples of the use of fat by different peoples in various parts of the world. Stefansson agrees with Dr Lutz about the impossibility of eating too much fat when this is not disguised in other foods, namely that overeating of fat per se induces vomiting.

CHAPTER 8

Page 172 *translated* This was work done by the author of this current book, who also helped Dr Lutz with the Synopsis, i.e. the summary of Life without Bread.

Page 172 *doses of cortisone* see Allan & Lutz p 36

Page 172 *my ideas on cancer* Please see chapter: 'Krebs' (cancer) pp 164-173 in the 14th edition of *Leben ohne Brot* (Lutz 1998), and Chapter Ten: 'Cancer: another Disease of Sugar Metabolism?' in *Life without Bread* (Allan & Lutz, 2000) p 163-178

Page 173 *pet formulas* All four doctors had their notions as to what this meant and their pet formulas as to how to translate this into practical advice for their patients! To Dr Lutz, this was an intake of carbohydrate in the region of 72g daily and with free choice as to protein and fat intake. To Blake Donaldson, it had meant half an hour's walk before breakfast and half a pound or so of fresh fat meat three times a day and a demitasse of black coffee. To Robert Atkins, it had meant a rather sudden cutting carbohydrate down to 15-20g a day until desired weight loss has been achieved, and then being guided by the stability of one's weight as to the establishing of a regular daily carbohydrate intake. To Dr Kwasniewski, the most suitable foods for our metabolism were eggs, followed by bone marrow and other food of animal origin; such food, he said, was a concentrated source of all necessary nutrients and so could be eaten in fairly small quantities, variety being largely unnecessary. These were the foundations to which they added their own details: for instance, the various amounts of vegetable matter and/or fruit, which might or might not be allowed.

Page 174 *enough amino acids* The quote comes from *Strong Medicine* p 43, with Donaldson maintaining the best source of the 10 essential amino acids, which are needed to grow and repair cells including those in our arteries, being fresh fat meat.

The colleagues mentioned here did not always stick to an all meat diet for their patients, sometimes allowing some plant food as an accompaniment to the meat. Donaldson found, for example, that some patients fared better when he added a limited amount of potato to their 8 oz meat and 2 oz fat three times daily.

Incidentally, Donaldson, Pennington and Thorpe openly acknowledged their debt to Stefansson, as did others in their circle of doctors in America at the time.

Page 184 *arteriosclerosis* Dr Lutz did acknowledge that it may not be carbohydrate consumption alone that contributed to the development of arteriosclerosis. In conversation, he mentioned that Greenlanders who were only eating 2% of carbohydrate in their diet sometimes developed arteriosclerosis in their old age. He wondered then about a connection between uric acid levels and arteriosclerosis.

Page 192 *Insulin resistance* has only relatively recently been recognised; it refers to when the cells no longer respond to insulin's instructions to admit more glucose and, as it were, shut their gates against it by closing receptors on the cell walls. When insulin resistance is combined with hyperinsulinism, the level of sugar in the blood and the urine rises: the first stage of diabetes.

Insulin resistance is a 'condition in which the body's ability of cells to use glucose properly is diminished' (Allan & Lutz p.33). The word 'properly' should be questioned, especially as insulin resistance is then described as a 'counter measure to excess insulin' in the same paragraph. In *Leben ohne Brot,* Dr Lutz himself talks of insulin resistance as an emergency brake: a defence mechanism on the part of the cells to protect themselves against the entry of too much sugar from the breakdown of carbohydrates.

Allan explains one of the main reasons why it is so important to keep sugar levels in the blood at relatively low levels throughout one's life and why the raised glucose levels in the blood and cells that comes with insulin resistance is so damaging to health:

> The answer lies in the chemistry and biochemistry of glucose and its interactions with proteins and lipids . . . glucose can react chemically [*glycation reactions*] with proteins to destroy their ability to function . . . Sugars that react in this way, such as glucose, are called *reducing sugars*. They can also react with lipids (fats) that make up cellular membranes. The higher the levels of sugar in our blood and tissues, the greater the chance that the destructive reactions between proteins, lipids and reducing sugars will take place. The process can eventually lead to the destruction of cellular function . . . it is normal for the sugar level to rise when a glucose load is given, but it should be removed from the blood within a few hours. The proper balance of sugar metabolism is what is needed to maintain good health. If you are continually snacking on carbohydrate foods, then sugar levels in the blood are always elevated.

> Allan & Lutz p 44–45

Page 193 *Lambarene* Here, Dr Albert Schweitzer established his hospital in the Central African Rainforest and it was here that he died at the age of 90 in 1965. When he first arrived, the indigenous population was largely living on a meagre diet of bananas and manioch root, with some meat when available. There was a lot of ill health, though no obvious cancer. Gradually, foods from the white traders entered their diet: tinned food (vegetables, meat and milk), tea and salt. See also Schweitzer (1929)

Page 193 *one explanation of cancer* This hypothesis, for which Dr Lutz acknowledges the work of Otto Warburg, who in turn drew on Louis Pasteur, was already expounded in the first edition of *Leben ohne Brot* (Lutz, 1967).

Berglas, in his General Summary and Conclusion, puts it this way:

It was shown that the biological import of pathological processes in general is to restore harmony in the disturbed organism and that carcinogenesis has to be interpreted as originating in a healing attempt on the part of the organism . . . The process of healing requires of the cells to become less differentiated and to return to the primitive state, and this must be considered the most important clue in understanding the process of cancer.

It was further shown that, when the healing process has been completed, the cells redifferentiate and are then again subject to the regulatory system of the organism. However, in the presence of chronic irritation, this process fails to be consummated. The cells remain dedifferentiated and gradually lose their power of redifferentiation. . . These now autonomous cells are then no longer controlled by the regulatory processes of the body, retaining only the functions of nutrition and reproduction essential to self-preservation. At this stage no further cellular irritation is required, the process then being irreversible – result: cancer.

We saw that not only benzpyrene, butter yellow etc., but also such diverse agents as glucose, viruses, bacteria, animal parasites, etc. can be cancer causing factors. The only thing common to all of them is their ability to produce chronic irritation. The so-called "carcinogens" merely differ in the rapidity of their action.

Berglas (1957) p.121

Note that Berglas, like Schole, sees glucose as a potentially cancer-promoting agent, an idea to which Dr Lutz paid special attention. Note, Berglas contended that 'cancer develops when the organism's regulatory mechanisms fail' (p xx, C3), and Allan talks of a 'consistent relationship between insulin resistance and many of our modern age-related diseases, including cancer' (Allan & Lutz Page 164).

Page 194 *cancer myself* Dr Lutz did not die of cancer; he was examined very fully at the end of his life but no cancer was found. He died at the age of 97 of a ruptured aortic aneurysm, an aneurysm which, according to medical colleagues, had been present for at least 10 years without giving trouble.

Page 196 *sanction obesity* If not, there has to be increased catabolism to help dispose of unwanted blood sugar. This was an area in which Dr Lutz could not quite see his way, and needs others to clarify.

CHAPTER 9

Page 204 *too little fat* It is interesting to note that even the UK Recommended Daily Intake (now called the Guideline Daily Amount and soon to be called the Reference Daily Intake) for fat is 70g for women, 95g for men and 70g for children 5-10 years. One wonders how many people deliberately following a low fat diet get even half this much?

Page 206 *tissue quality* Several reasons are given for the diminished tissue quality that seems to accompany carbohydrate overload. The contribution made by the diminished action of the growth hormone has already been mentioned.

Dr Lutz also talks of the too frequent need for gluconeogenesis and postulates a type of night-starvation in those eating high levels of carbohydrate. Gluconeogenesis is the synthesising of blood sugar from non-carbohydrate sources, sometimes including the breaking down of the body's own protein for example from the musculature, as happens for instance in starvation (*Leben ohne Brot* 16th edition, pp 43–4).

A further reason lies in the damage to body tissues from glycation reactions, explained by Allan (see above p 245).

Page 208 *epilepsy* In his first book, Dr Lutz says he got very encouraging results treating young epileptics, often achieving a complete freedom from attacks or at least a lessening of their incidence; he speaks of these patients being 'kohlenhydratfrei' (carbohydrate-free), by which he tends to mean low carbohydrate but grain-free (*Leben ohne Brot* 1967). His work with epilepsy was mainly done before he moved to Salzburg in 1968 and the actual amount of carbohydrate Dr Lutz used is not specified. In later editions of his book, he urges doctors to consider a ketogenic diet for epileptic patients: this suggests that, in the early days of his practice, Dr Lutz had been using the very low carbohydrate diet which he was initially using for his patients with multiple sclerosis, perhaps 10–20g of carbohydrate. There is also mention of older patients who profited thereby.

A ketogenic diet, sometimes seen as a starvation diet, is one in which the carbohydrate content is so low that the brain derives its energy from fat (ketone bodies derived from the breakdown of fatty acids) rather than glucose. Dr Lutz did not consider his more liberal diet of 72g as ketogenic, for which he thought it necessary to eat less than 60g carbohydrate daily.

Page 209 *allergic to* In general, allergy did not form part of Dr Lutz's repertoire. When I asked him about this, he said he had no experience of dealing with allergies as such but that some of his patients reported that, after a while on his diet, though their main long-term allergies persisted, peripheral recently acquired allergic reactions had ceased.

Page 210 *related to arteriosclerosis* See the section on Alzheimer's in the 14th edition of *Leben ohne Brot* for more technical details of the similarities.

Page 216 *brain-worker* This question was raised shortly after Dr Lutz's first book was published and gave rise to an interchange of letters between J Kühnau (1968) and himself (1969) in the *Deutsche med. Wochenschrift.*

Page 216 *from fat* See Allan and Lutz for an explanation of this procedure.

Page 226 *other serious health problems* Dr Lutz sees a whole wide range of conditions as very probably influenced or induced (directly or indirectly, partly or wholly) by the effects of excessive carbohydrate consumption. Among very many, he lists rickets (which he says is certainly not caused by vitamin D deficiency alone), osteomalacia and other bone problems such as scoliosis and Scheuermann's disease, various weaknesses of muscles and ligaments, splay and flat feet. He also mentions that problems of ageing are speeded up by tissue loss or damage: loss of muscle, periodontal disease, emphysema, arteriosclerosis, disorders of the heart muscle, age-related brain damage and so on. See, for example, what Dr Lutz calls the 'protein sacrifice' in Dismantling a Myth pp 90–92.

Page 230 *wittingly or not* The Diabetes UK still advises a low fat diet + their GDA lists calories, fat, salt and fibre, states that 50% of calories are to be derived from carbohydrate but omits specifying a suitable amount for diabetics; the 2014 UK general Guideline Daily Amount is for a carbohydrate intake of 220 g for children of 5-10 years, 230 g for women and 300 g for men, that is three to four times the amount of carbohydrate that Dr Lutz saw as the amount best suited for the maintenance of all-round, long-term health.

REFERENCES

AHRENS E H (1979), 'Dietary Fats and Coronary Heart Disease: Unfinished Business', *The Lancet*, December 22/29

ALLAN C, LUTZ W J (2000), *Life without Bread: How a Low-Carbohydrate Diet Can Save Your Life*, Keats, USA

ATKINS R C (1972), *Dr Atkins' Diet Revolution*, Bantam Books, N Y

ATKINS R, GARE G (1994), *Dr Atkins' New Diet Cookbook*, M Evans & Co, New York

BERGLAS A (1957), *Cancer, nature, cause and cure*, Institute Pasteur

BRACKEN V (2013), *Uncle Wolfi's Secret*, Just Perhaps? Edinburgh

BRONOWSKI J (1979), *The Ascent of Man*, BBC Publications, London, p 64

CHORLTON W (1983), *Ice Ages*, Planet Earth Series, Time-Life Books Inc., Alexandria, Virginia, pp 24–30

CLEAVE C L (1974), *The Saccharine Diseases*, John Wright & Sons, Bristol

DONALDSON B (1963), *Strong Medicine*, Cassell & Co Ltd, London

DRAPER H H, 'Nutrition Studies: The Aboriginal Eskimo Diet – A modern Perspective', *The Eskimo of Northwestern Alaska: A biological Perspective*, JAMISON, ZEGURA & MILAN (1978)

ECKEL K, LUTZ W (1961), 'Über die Behandlung der Multiple Sklerose mittels Kohlenhydratentzuges', *Wien. klin. Wschr.*, pp 493–5

FOLEY R (1997), *Humans before Humanity*, Blackwell Publishers, Oxford

GLATZEL H (1974), 'Sinn und Unsinn in der Diätetik', VIII Ischämie, Herzkrankheiten, *Med. Welt* 25, 116

GLATZEL H, Foreword to the Fifth Edition, *Leben ohne Brot* LUTZ (1975)

GLATZEL H (1982), *Wege und Irrwege moderner Ernährung*, Hippokrates Verlag, Stuttgart

GORDON T (1971), *The Framingham Diet Study*, Section 24 'Diet and the Regulation of Serum Cholesterol', US Govt Printing Office

HEILMEYER L (1953), 'Allgemeine klinische Bedeutung des Hypophysen-Nebenierenrindensystems' *Probleme des Hypophysen Nebenierenrinden- systems*, WEISSBECKER, Springer-Verlag, Berlin

HAAS L (1984), *Der Einfluss different gestalteter Kohlenhydrat-Fett-Diäten auf die Inzidenz Axoymethan-induzierter Tumoren bei Ratten*, Dissertation, Tierärztliche Hochschule, Hannover

HEATON K W (1973), 'Food fibre as an obstacle to energy intake', *The Lancet*, Vol. 2, Pt 7843, pp 1418–1421

HERODOTUS (translated DE SELINCOURT A, 1954), *Herodotus: The histories* (III/2), Penguin Classics

JAMESON G, WILLIAMS E (1964), *The Drinking Man's Diet*, Cameron & Co, San Francisco

JAMISON P L, ZEGURA S L, MILAN F A (1978), *The Eskimo of Northwestern Alaska: A biological Perspective*, Dowden, Hutchinson and Ross, Stroudsburg, Pennsylvania

KASPER H, LUTZ W, WILD M (1979), 'Die Höhe der Nährstoff-, Cholesterin- und Ballaststoffzufuhr unter kohlenhydratarmer Diät bei freier Wahl der Fett- und Proteinzufuhr', *Aktuelle Ernährung* 4, 155–157

KAUNITZ H (1976), 'Sind die Nahrungsfette bei der Arteriosklerose von spezifischer Bedeutung?' *Münch. med. Wschr.* 119, 539

KAUNITZ, H (1978), 'Cholesterol & Repair Process in Arteriosclerosis', *Lipids* Vol. 13, Nr 5, 373–374

REFERENCES

KÜHN H (1954), *Das Erwachen der Menschheit*, Fischer Bücherei, Frankfurt-M / Hamburg

KÜHNAU J (1968), 'Leben ohne Brot?', *Dtsch. med. Wschr.* 93, 2089

KWASNIEWSKI J with CHYLINSKI M (1999), *Die optimale Ernährung*, Zuber, Vienna

LIEB C W (1926), 'The Effects of an Exclusive, Long-Continued Meat Diet', *J. A. M. A.*, July 3

LIEB C W (1929), 'The Effects on Human Beings of a Twelve Months' exclusive Meat Diet', *J. A. M. A.*, July 6

LIEB C W (1935), 'A Year's Exclusive Meat Diet and Seven Years Later', *Am. J. of Digestive Diseases and Nutrition*, Vol. 2, 8

LORENZ-MEYER H, BAUER P et al (1996), *Scand. J. of Gastroenterology*, 31, 778

LUNDBAEK et al, (1972), 'Anxiety, Growth Hormone and Glucose Tolerance in Normal Children', *Acta med. scand.*, 192, pp 539–542

LUTZ W, ISELSTÖGER H (1960), 'Veränderungen der Sexualhormonausscheidung im Harn auf Kohlenhydratentzug', *Münchener med. Wschr.* 102, pp 1963–5

LUTZ W (1962), 'Vier Jahre ohne Kohlenhydrate', *Medizin und Ernährung*, 3 Jhrg. Nr.3

LUTZ W (1962), 'Arteriosclerose und Kohlenhydrate?', *Wiener Z. Innere Medizin*, 1

LUTZ W J (1964), 'Das endocrine Syndrom des adipösen Jugendlichen', *Wiener med. Wsch.*, 451

LUTZ W (1965), 'Die Behandlung der Colitis ulcerosa durch Entzug von Kohlenhydraten', *Wiener med. Wochenschrift*, 25/26,

LUTZ W (1967), 'Die Behandlung der Colitis ulcerosa durch Kohenhydratbeschränkung – Bericht über 40 Fälle', *Wiener med. Wochenschrift*, 660

LUTZ W (1967), *Leben ohne Brot*, Selecta Verlag, Planegg bei München

LUTZ W (1968), 'Kohlenhydratabhängig Polyglobulie', *Wiener med. Wochenschrift*, 583

LUTZ W (1969), *Dtsch. med. Wschr.* 94, 338

LUTZ W J, ANDRESEN G, BUDDECKE E (1969), 'Untersuchungen über den Einfluss einer kohlenhydratarmen Langzeitdiät auf die Arteriosklerose des Huhnes', *Zeitschrift für Ernährungswissenschaft* 9, 222.

LUTZ W (1970), *Internistischer Alltag,* Selecta-Verlag, Munich

LUTZ W (1975), 'Pathologische Lebertests unter Kohlenhydratarmen Diät', *Wiener med. Wochenschrift*, 125, pp 292–5

LUTZ W (1976), 'Hypo- und hypersiderosen unter Kohlenhydratarmer Diät', *Wiener med. Wschr.*, 126, pp 221–4

LUTZ W (1977), Ernährung und Risikofaktoren, *Wiener medizinische Wochenschrift*, 127

LUTZ W (1981), 'Low-carbohydrate Diet in Ulcerative.Colitis and Crohn's Disease', *Coloproctology* III, 349

LUTZ W (1985), 'Morbus Crohn unter kohlenhydratarmer Diät', *Coloproctology*, 278

LUTZ W (1985), 'Morbus Crohn, eine allergische Reaktion auf resorbierte Makropartikel?', *Deutsche med. Wochenschrift*, 1394

LUTZ W (1986), *Die Lutz Diät,* Ariston Verlag, Geneva

LUTZ W (1986), *Dismantling a Myth: the Role of Fat and Carbohydrates in our Diet,* Charles Thomas, Springfield, USA, and Selecta-Verlag, Munich

LUTZ W (1987), 'Morbus Crohn unter kohlenhydratarmer Diät, Langzeitbeobachtung an 67 Fällen', *Münchener medizinische Wochenschrift*, 921

LUTZ W (1988), *Cholesterin und tierische Fette,* SMV Edition Materia Medica, Munich

LUTZ W (1989), 'Arteriosklerose und Krebs – Fette oder Kohlenhydrate?', *Wiener klin. Wschr.*, 9 June, pp 429–433

REFERENCES

LUTZ W (1995), *Kranker Magen kranker Darm: Was wirklich hilft,* SAYLA Fachverlag Gmbh, Gräfelfing

LUTZ W J (1995), 'The Colonisation of Europe and our Western Diseases', *Medical Hypothesis* 45, pp 115–120

LUTZ W J (1998), *Leben ohne Brot,* 14th edition, INFORMED, Gräfelfing

LUTZ W (1998), *Life without bread: a synopsis,* published privately

MACKARNESS R (1958), *Eat Fat and Grow Slim,* Harvill Press, reprinted Fontana Books 1961 (Doubleday and Co, New York)

MACKARNESS R (1976), *Not All in the Mind,* Pan Books Ltd p 54

McCARRISON Sir R (1982), *Nutrition and Health,* The McCarrison Society, London

McCLELLAN W S, DU BOIS E F (1930), 'Prolonged meat diets with a study of kidney function and ketosis', *Journal of Biol. Chemistry,* July, 651 – 668

McGREW W C (1992), *Chimpanzee Material Culture – Implications for Human Evolution,* Cambridge University Press

MANN G V (1977), 'Diet Heart, End of an Era', *New Engl. J. Med.* 297 p 644

MANN G V (1993), *Coronary Heart Disease: the dietary sense and nonsense,* Janus Publishing Co, London

MOHLER H (1978), *Die Cholesterin-Neurose,* Otto Salle Verlag Frankfurt/Main

OLSON R E (1980), 'Toward Healthful Diets', *Report to the US-Academy of Science,* April, p 28

OLIVER M (1983), 'Should we not forget about mass control of coronary risk factors?', *Lancet* II, p 37

PAULITSCHKO R (1986), Report on my illness: ulcerative colitis / morbus Crohn, and their healing, unpublished manuscript

PENNINGTON A W (1953), 'A reorientation on obesity', *New England Journal of Medicine,* vol. 248, no. 23

PENNINGTON A W (1954), 'Treatment of obesity: Developments of the past 150 years', *American Journal of Digestive Diseases*, March

PRICE W (1998), *Nutrition and Physical Degeneration*, Keats, USA

REAVEN G M (1976), *Commentary*, Palo Alto Veterans Administration

SALLMAN H., HARISCH G., SCHOLE J. (1976), 'Über den Einfluss einer kohlenhydratarmen Langzeitdiät auf die Arteriosklerose des Huhnes', *Zbl. Vet. Med.* A 23, pp 635–644

SANDARS N K (1972) translator, *The Epic of Gilgamesh*, Penguin Books, Harmondsworth, England

SCHOLE J (1972), 'Nahrungsfett aus der Sicht der Ernährungs-endokrinologie', *Symposium presentation*, Munich

SCHOLE J, HARISCH G, SALLMANN H P (1978), *Belastung, Ernährung und Resistenz*, Verlag Paul Parey, Hamburg, Berlin

SCHOLE J, 'Foreword to ninth German edition of *Leben ohne Brot*', translated in *Dismantling a Myth*, LUTZ (1986), pp 10–11

SCHOLE J, LUTZ W J (1988), *Regulationskrankheiten*, F.Enke, Stuttgart

SCHWEITZER A (1929), *On the Edge of the Primeval Forest*, A & C Black Ltd, London

SCHWEITZER A, Preface to *Cancer, Nature and Cure*, BERGLAS (1957)

SELYE H (1936), 'A syndrome produced by diverse nocuous agents', *Nature*, 4 July

SELYE H (1946), 'The general adaptation syndrome and the diseases of adaptation', *The Journal of Allergy*, Vol. 17, July/Sept/Nov

SELYE H (1952), *The Story of the Adaptation Syndrome*, Acta Inc., Montreal

STEFANNSON V (1913), *My Life with the Eskimo*, reprinted 1951, MACMILLAN

STEFANNSON V (1918), 'Observations on Three Cases of Scurvy', *Jnal of American Medical Association*, Nov. 23

REFERENCES

STEFANNSON V (1921), *The Friendly Arctic,* MACMILLAN, New York

STEFANNSON V (1935–6), 'Adventures in Diet', *Harper's Monthly Magazine,* Nov, p 668, Dec, p 46, Jan, p 178

STEFANSSON V (1946), *Not by Bread Alone,* MACMILLAN, N Y, pp 5–6

STEFANSSON V (1953), *The Friendly Arctic,* MACMILLAN, N Y, p 610

STEFANSSON V (1956), *The Fat of the Land,* MACMILLAN

STEFANSSON V (1960), *Cancer: Disease of Civilisation,* Hill and Wang, New York

STEFANSSON V (1964), *Discovery,* McGraw-Hill Book Company, New York, pp 385–386

STEHBENS W, 'The Pathology of Atherosclerosis', *Coronary Heart Disease: the dietary sense and nonsense,* MANN (1993)

STOUT R W & VALLANCE-OWEN (1969), 'Insulin and Atheroma', *The Lancet,* May 31

SYKES B (2001), *The Seven Daughters of Eve,* Bantam Press pp 1–2

THORPE G L (1957), 'Treating overweight patients', *J. Am. Med. Assoc.,* vol. 165, no. 11, pp 1361–5

TOLSTOI E (1929), 'The effect of an exclusive meat diet lasting one year on the carbohydrate tolerance of two normal men', *Journal of Biological Chemistry,* Sept, pp 747–752

TORREY J C, MONTU E (1931), 'The influence of an exclusive meat diet on the flora of the human colon', *Journal of Infectious Diseases,* August, pp 141–176

WEITZEL G, BUDDECKE E I (1956), *Klin. Wschr.* 34, 1171

WEITZEL G, Preface, *Leben ohne Brot* LUTZ (1967)

YELLOWLEES W (1993), *A Doctor in the Wilderness,* Janus Publishing Co, London, p 147

YUDKIN J (1971), 'Ernährung und Atherosklerose', *Med. und Ernährung* 12

FURTHER PUBLICATIONS:
Dr med. habil. Wolfgang Lutz

1938 'Über einen neuen Weg zum Nachweis jodhaltiger Kontrastmittel usw', (with H Seyfried), *Klinische Wochenschrift*, 908

1938 'Zur Wertung der oralen Cholezystographie', *Klin. Wochenschrift*, 933

1938 'Gefahren der intravenösen Cholezystographie', (with H Seyfried), *Münchener med. Wochenschrift*, 1019

1938 'Über die Resorption von oral verabreichtem Tetrajodphenolphthalein', *Klinische Wochenschrift*, 1180

1939 'Der Einfluss von Galle und gallensauren Salzen auf die Resorption von Totrajodphenolphthalein', (with H Seyfried), *Wiener klin. Wschr.*, 10

1939 'Leberzelleistung und enterohepatischer Kreislauf', *Wiener klinische Wochenschrift*, 25

1939 'Ulironbstimmung nach Hecht in Stufenphotometer', *Klinische Wochenschrift*, 996

1939 'Über die Bedeutung der Galle für Resorption und Ausscheidung von Uliron', *Klinische Wochenschrift*, 967

1942 'Die Überlebenszeit nach Drucksturz in grössten Höhen', *Luftfahrtmedizin*, 7, 1.

1942 'Tierversuche zum Fallschirmabsprung aus Überdruckkabinen', (with H J Wendt), *Mitteilungen aus dem Gebiet der Luftfahrtmedizin*, 1, *Geheimbericht an das deutsche Luftfahrtministerium*

1943 'Der anoxische Scheintod', *Luftfahrtmedizin*, 171

1943 'Über die Wirkung von Kohlensäure auf die Erholung aus Sauerstoff- mangel' (with H J Wendt, V Werz, H Zirngibl), *Luftfahrtmedizin*, 249

1943 'Die experimentelle Verkaltbüterung des Warmblüters', *Klin. Wschr.* 727

1944 'Elektrokardiographische Beobachtungen bei Auskühlung des Warmblüters', *Z. Kreislaufforschung*, 22—24

1944 'Kältetod und Sauerstoffmangel', (with R von Werz), Münchener med. Wochenschrift

1948 'Zur Temperaturabhängigkeit der Erregungsvorganges im Herzen', *Zeitschrift für Kreislaufforschung*, 9, 10

1948 'Über Wesen und Ursache des Herzstillstandes bei Auskühlung', *Zeitschrift für Kreislaufforschung*, 11, 12

1949 'Die Depressionsatelektase', *Wiener Z. Innere Med.*

1949 'Neue Wege bei der Wiederbelebung Erfrorener', *Wiener med. Wochenschrift*, 99, 287

1950 'Kältetod und Wiederbelebung', *Archiv für innere Medizin*, 1, 470

1951 'Die Bedeutung der künstlichen Atmung für die Wiederbelebung nach tiefer Auskühlung', *Wiener Z. Innere Med.*, 32, 36

1951 'Leben bei niedriger Körpertemperatur', (with R von Werz)., *Münchener med. Wochenschrift*, 93

1951 'Achylische Kardiopathie', *Wiener Z. Innere Med.*, 10, 32

1952 'Der röntgenkymographische Ausdruck des venösen Windkessels', *Z. Kreislauf*, 3, 4

1952 'Der Wert des Prostigmintestes für die Pancreasdiagnostik', *Wiener med. Wochenschrift*, 26, 27

1953 'Die therapeutische Wirkung intravenöser Kleindosen von ACTH', (with O Metzenroth), *Wiener med. Wochenschrift*, 25, 26

1953 'Die experimentellen Grundlagen der Kältenarkose', *Der Anästhesist*, Bd 2, Heft 5

1953 'Experimentelle Untersuchungen zur Behandlung der Luftembolie mit erhöhtem Atmosphärendruck', *Der Anästhesist*, Bd 2, Heft 6

1955 'Veränderungen des pathologischen EKC auf ACTH', *Kreislaufforschung*, 221

1954 'Ein vereinfachter 'Thorn' Test', *Münchener med. Wochenschrift*, 34

1957 'Plazenta-Extrakt und Eosinophilen-Reaktion', *Med. Klinik*, 1B

1959 'Kältetod und Kàltenarkose', *Die Kälte*, 10

1959 'Die Überwindung des Kältetodes', *Z. gesamte experimentelle Medizin* Bd. 115, 615-637

1969 'Diätetische Therapie der Arteriosklerose, *Wiener klin. Wschr.*, 466

1971 'Umrisse einer neuen Ernährungslehre', *Österreichische Ärztezeitung*, 3, 212

1972 'Zum Problem der kohlenhydratarmen Ernährung', *Therapie der Gegenwart*, 111, 367, 514

1975 'Carbohydrates and Disease', *Morristown Memorial Hospital Journal*, 1, 4–10 Oct.

1977 'Kohlenhydratarme Diät', *Deutsche med. Wochenschrift*, 6, 212

1977 'Which diet?', *Nature*, 270

1979 'Kohlenhydratarme Diät bei Colitis ulcerosa', *Münchener med. Wochenschrift*, 953

1979 'Influence of Different Diets on Growth and Serum Composition of Japanese Quail', (With Cihak, Peter and Hesse), *Zool. J. Physiol.*, 83, 149

1980 'Die Kohlenhydrattheorie der Arteriosklerose, *Wiener med. Wochenschrift*, 625

1981 'Bemerkung zur Arbeit von J W Brandes und H Lorenz-Meyer Zuckerfreie Diät, eine neue Perspektive zur Behandlung des Morbus Crohn?', *Z. Gastroenterologie*, 1–12

1981 'Multiple Sclerose, *Deutsche med. Wochenschrift*, 221

1981 'Diätetische und medikamentöse Therapie der Zerebralsklerose', *Therapiewoche*, 31, 7406

1984 'Tonsillektomie bei Kindern', *Deutsche klin. Wochenschrift* 37, 1424

1991 'Lebenserwartung – was ist mit den Japanern los?, *Wiener med. Wochenschrift*, 148

1994 'Die Kohlenhydrat-Theorie', *Wiener med. Wochenschrift*, 144, 387

1996 'Die Lipid-Theorie kommt in die Jahre', *J. Cardiol.*, 94

INDEX

Printed in Great Britain
by Amazon